Fats.

They're the black-hatted bad guys of nutrition, the most demonized of all nutrients. Even the word *fat* itself conjures up all sorts of negative associations when used in everyday language. Take the expressions *fathead, fat chance, fat cat,* or *fatso,* for example. *Fat* is practically a four-letter word.

But is fat really all that bad? Does it deserve to be so maligned?

This may come as a surprise to you, but fats are mostly good guys in nutrition . . .

Other Books by the Author

WRINKLE-FREE:
YOUR GUIDE TO YOUTHFUL SKIN AT ANY AGE

THE BONE DENSITY TEST

THE CELLULITE BREAKTHROUGH

HAIR SAVERS FOR WOMEN:
A COMPLETE GUIDE TO TREATING AND PREVENTING HAIR LOSS

NATURAL WEIGHT LOSS MIRACLES

21 DAYS TO BETTER FITNESS

KAVA:
THE ULTIMATE GUIDE TO NATURE'S ANTI-STRESS HERB

Other Books Coauthored by the Author

LEAN BODIES

LEAN BODIES TOTAL FITNESS

30 DAYS TO SWIMSUIT LEAN

HIGH PERFORMANCE NUTRITION

POWER EATING

SHAPE TRAINING

HIGH PERFORMANCE BODYBUILDING

50 WORKOUT SECRETS

BUILT! THE NEW BODYBUILDING FOR EVERYONE

good fat

vs.

BAD FAT

Maggie Greenwood-Robinson, Ph.D.

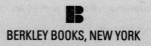

BERKLEY BOOKS, NEW YORK

Note: Every effort has been made to ensure that the information contained in this book is complete and accurate. However, neither the publisher nor the author is engaged in rendering professional advice or services to the individual reader. The ideas, procedures, and suggestions contained in this book are not intended as a substitute for consulting with your physician. All matters regarding your health require medical supervision. Neither the author nor the publisher shall be liable or responsible for any loss, injury, or damage allegedly arising from any information or suggestion in this book. The opinions expressed in this book represent the personal views of the author and not of the publisher.

GOOD FAT VS. BAD FAT

A Berkley Book / published by arrangement with
the author

PRINTING HISTORY
Berkley edition / January 2002

All rights reserved.
Copyright © 2002 by Maggie Greenwood-Robinson, Ph.D.
Book design by Kristin del Rosario
Cover design by Rita Frangie
This book, or parts thereof, may not be reproduced in
any form without permission.
For information address:
The Berkley Publishing Group, a division of Penguin Putnam Inc.,
375 Hudson Street, New York, New York 10014.

Visit our website at
www.penguinputnam.com

ISBN: 0-425-18427-7

BERKLEY®
Berkley Books are published by The Berkley Publishing Group,
a division of Penguin Putnam Inc., 375 Hudson Street,
New York, New York 10014.
BERKLEY and the "B" design
are trademarks belonging to Penguin Putnam Inc.

PRINTED IN THE UNITED STATES OF AMERICA

10 9 8 7 6 5

To my brother Tom and my sister Gretchen, with love

CONTENTS

Part IV. The Fat-Burning Fats

Part V. Designing a Fat-Healthy Diet

ACKNOWLEDGMENTS

I gratefully thank the following people for their work and contributions to this book: my agent Madeleine Morel, 2M Communications, Ltd.; Christine Zika and the staff at The Berkley Publishing Group; and my husband, Jeff, for love and patience during the research and writing of this book.

PART I

Fats:
The Good, the Bad, and the Ugly

ONE

The Fats of Life

Fats.

They're the black-hatted bad guys of nutrition, the most demonized of all nutrients. Even the word *fat* itself conjures up all sorts of negative associations when used in everyday language. Take the expressions *fathead, fat chance, fat cat,* and *fatso,* for example. *Fat* is practically a four-letter word.

But is fat really all that bad? Does it deserve to be so maligned?

This may come as a surprise to you, but fats are mostly good guys in nutrition. You need them to survive. In fact, there are a slew of "good" fats with astonishing powers to outwit disease and keep you healthy for a lifetime. Sure, there are some health-risky fats, but even some of those are needed in small amounts for good health. When you're dealing with fats, the key is to control not only the amount you eat but also the kind of fat you eat.

To get a handle on how fats affect your health, it helps to learn some basic facts about this most misunderstood of all nutrients. So let's get started on a short nutrition lesson.

FAT FACTS

You've heard the old expression, "Oil and water don't mix." Well, fats—many of which are oils—are members of a family of chemical compounds technically known as *lipids* that for the most part don't dissolve in water. You know this if you've ever made salad dressing and watched the fatty part separate from the rest of the liquid and gradually rise to the top.

When we speak of fat in our foods or on our bodies, we're talking about *triglycerides.* Triglycerides make up about 95 percent of dietary fat and 90 percent of body fat. Some triglycerides also circulate in your bloodstream. Chemically, a triglyceride is a backbone of glycerol (a type of alcohol) to which three fatty acids are attached, hence the name triglyceride.

A *fatty acid* is a building block of fat. Many specific types of fatty acids are found in various fats, each with different properties that influence your health in farreaching ways. Fatty acids are contructed of chains of carbon atoms with hydrogen atoms attached, with an acid group at one end. Think of this configuration as a charm bracelet. The carbons form the chain, and the hydrogen and the acid group are the charms.

The lengths of these chains vary according to the fat. Fats found in meat, for example, usually have chains that are sixteen or more carbons long. Some carbon chains are much shorter, with six, eight, ten, or twelve carbon atoms.

Is the length of a fat chain important?

Yes. Here's the deal: Length has a lot to do with how

your body uses the fat and obtains energy from it. Short-
and medium-chain fatty acids, which are generally found
in butter and coconut oil, are a good example. During
digestion, they are absorbed more readily by your body
than longer-chain fatty acids are and thus supply quick
energy. Because of this, short- and medium-chain fatty
acids are less likely to be packed away as body fat.
Longer-chain fatty acids, on the other hand, tend to be
stored as fat. So to a certain extent, length matters.

Saturated and Unsaturated Fatty Acids

Fatty acids from food are chemically classified not only
by the length of their chains but also according to the
number of hydrogens the fatty acid chain holds. This attribute is referred to as *saturation.*

When a fatty acid carries the maximum number of hydrogen atoms, it is said to be loaded or *saturated.* If there
are one or more places in the chain where hydrogens are
missing, the fatty acid is *unsaturated.* A fatty acid with a
single point of unsaturation is termed *monounsaturated;*
a fatty acid with two or more points is called *polyunsaturated.*

The degree of saturation affects the temperature at
which the fat melts. Generally speaking, the more saturated the fatty acids of a fat are, the more solid the fat is
at room temperature. Examples of saturated fats include
those found in beef, butter, lard, and dairy products. Unsaturated fats such as vegetable oils are usually liquid at
room temperature. An exception to the rule that saturated
fats are more solid than unsaturated fats is coconut oil, a
saturated fat that is liquid at room temperature.

Monounsaturated fatty acids, a type of unsaturated fat,
are found in such foods as olive oil, olives, avocado,

cashew nuts, and cold-water fish such as salmon, mackerel, halibut, and swordfish. The most common monounsaturated fatty acid in our food is oleic acid, a major
component of olive oil. Monounsaturated fats are generally liquid at room temperature but will partially solidify
when refrigerated.

The other type of unsaturated fat is polyunsaturated fat.
Found in fish and in most vegetable oils, these foods are
endowed with vitaminlike nutrients known as essential
fatty acids (EFAs) that your body needs for normal cell
growth and development. EFAs are so important that they
deserve further explanation (see the next section).

Some polyunsaturated fats such as shortening and stick
margarine are hard at room temperature, but only because
they have undergone a process called *hydrogenation,*
which solidifies vegetable oils.

All fats, whether of vegetable origin or animal origin,
feature some combination of saturated fatty acids, monounsaturated fatty acids, and polyunsaturated fatty acids.
Animal fats, for example, contain about 50 percent saturated fat, while most vegetable fats are predominantly
polyunsaturated fatty acids.

A myth exists that saturated fats contain more calories
than either polyunsaturated or monounsaturated fats do.
Not so. All pure fats yield 9 calories per gram, and about
115 to 120 calories per tablespoon. However, there may
be a slight variation in calories depending on whether the
fat is solid or liquid. Solid fats such as butter or margarine
contain some air or water and thus will not have as many
calories as the same amount of oil. Reduced-calorie or
imitation margarines have even fewer calories because
they contain more water.

Essential Fatty Acids

Your body can make nearly all the fatty acids it needs for good health—with the exception of essential fatty acids (EFAs), which must be supplied by your diet. Found in plant oils and fish, EFAs are polyunsaturated fats that regulate an amazing number of cellular processes and are endowed with an impressive list of life-sustaining benefits. More than sixty health problems, from heart disease to inflammatory illnesses to immune disorders, can be treated with EFAs.

Unfortunately, though, about 80 percent of all Americans are deficient in these vital nutrients. A major reason is that most of the fat in our diets has been refined and chemically altered—and, in the process, stripped of its essential fatty acids. Examples of synthetic fats include hydrogenated fats and trans-fatty acids found in shortening, stick margarine, fast foods, and commercially baked products such as crackers and cookies. Trans-fatty acids, in particular, can make up to 5 to 35 percent of the fat in margarines, shortenings, and other hydrogenated fats.

Like two riders trying to hop into the same taxi, synthetic fats compete with essential fatty acids for entry into your metabolic pathways, with processed fats muscling essential fats out of the way most of the time. This metabolic mix-up undermines the healing power of essential fatty acids.

How Do EFAs Work?

In actuality, just two fatty acids are considered "essential": linoleic acid (LA) and alpha-linolenic acid (ALA). Both are required for normal cell structure and function. Basically, they make cell membranes more permeable so that nutrient-carrying fluids can pass into cells and waste materials can leave. By contrast, saturated fats stiffen the membranes of cells, making them impermeable and jeopardizing the health of the cells. Thus, it's vital to consume adequate amounts of linoleic acid and alpha-linolenic acid in your diet every day.

Found mostly in vegetable oils, nuts, seeds, and margarine, linoleic acid helps transport water across the skin and ensures the proper functioning of the pituitary gland, which is involved in growth. These actions make linoleic acid a good treatment for skin problems, as well as a potentially therapeutic agent in growth and development therapies. Available from fish, flaxseed oil, and other vegetable oils, alpha-linoleic acid has been studied for its role in fighting heart disease, stroke, and many other serious illnesses.

Both of these essential fatty acids act as "parents," giving birth to other fatty acids in a process involving enzymes. For instance, alpha-linolenic acid produces two fatty acids that play various health-enhancing roles in the body: eicosapentaenoic acid (EPA) and docosahexaenoic acid (DHA). EPA is a very potent fatty acid that prevents platelets in the blood from abnormal clotting, and it helps reduce inflammation. DHA is an important constituent of the brain and retina. Although your body makes DHA and EPA from alpha-linolenic acid, you can obtain them directly from fish in your diet.

Linoleic acid produces gamma-linolenic acid (GLA), which is converted to dihomo-gamma-linoleic acid (DGLA), and then to arachidonic acid (AA). GLA, in particular, has far-reaching benefits in treating all sorts of diseases, particularly those involving inflammation.

In addition to being synthesized from linoleic acid, arachidonic acid occurs naturally in animal and plant foods. Although necessary for infant brain development, arachidonic acid can be harmful in excessive amounts. Arachidonic acid counters the positive action of eicosapentaenoic acid. For instance, if a platelet has a lot of arachidonic acid in its cell membrane, it will clot more readily. On the other hand, a platelet is less likely to clot if there is a lot of eicosapentaenoic acid in its membrane.

These offspring, or derivative, fatty acids manufacture hormonelike compounds called eicosanoids, which include prostaglandins and leukotrienes. Responsible for many of the healing properties of essential fatty acids, prostaglandins and leukotrienes regulate numerous processes, including blood pressure, normal blood clot formation, blood lipids, immunity, inflammation in response to injury, and many other vital functions.

There are "good" prostaglandins and "bad" prostaglandins. Similarly, there are "less inflammatory" leukotrienes and "pro-inflammatory" leukotrienes. A series of good prostaglandins called prostaglandins 1 (PGE1) are synthesized from DGLA. The job of PGE1 is to reduce inflammation, dilate blood vessels, and inhibit blood clotting.

Another series of good prostaglandins called prostaglandins 3 (PGE3) are derived from EPA. So are the less inflammatory leukotrienes. PGE3 helps your body fight infection.

A group of bad prostaglandins called prostaglandins 2 (PGE2), as well as the pro-inflammatory leukotrienes, is synthesized from arachidonic acid. PGE2 steps up inflammation, constricts blood vessels, and encourages abnormal blood clotting.

It's important to understand these metabolic processes. By altering the type of essential fat you eat, you can manipulate the levels of these eicosanoids in your body to treat inflammation, allergies, high blood pressure, and many other adverse health conditions.

Here's how: It's desirable to reduce levels of arachidonic acid and increase DGLA and EPA. This gives rise to more good prostaglandins and leukotrienes. You can accomplish this goal by cutting back on saturated fats (which encourage the production of arachidonic acid), eating more fish (which is loaded with EPA), and supplementing your diet with vegetable oils high in alpha-linolenic acid such as flaxseed oil.

Generally speaking, your body strives to strike a delicate balance among PGE1, PGE2, PGE3, and the leukotrienes. But unless enough of the good prostaglandins are produced, the bad prostaglandins will gang up on your system and harm your body.

Table 1 illustrates how the essential fatty acids are ultimately converted into prostaglandins and leukotrienes.

What Are Omega Fats?

No doubt, you have heard the term *omega fats* used to describe different types of fats. This is simply another classification of essential fatty acids. The omega-3 fatty acids include alpha-linolenic acid (ALA) and its derivative fatty acids, eicosapentaenoic acid (EPA) and docosahexaenoic acid (DHA). The main omega-6 fatty acids are linoleic acid (LA) and its derivative fatty acids, gamma-linolenic acid (GLA) and arachidonic acid (AA). (The designations 3 and 6 refer to their molecular structures.)

Omega-3 fatty acids are vital for normal growth and development and may play a key role in preventing and treating heart disease, high blood pressure, diabetes, arthritis, and cancer. Omega-6 fatty acids are generally nec-

Table 1

ESSENTIAL FATTY ACID METABOLISM

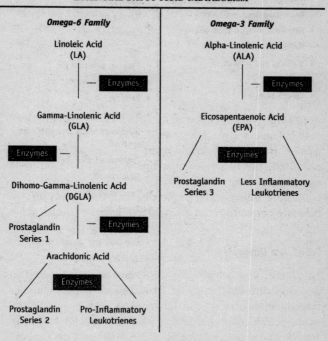

Omega-6 Family	Omega-3 Family
Linoleic Acid (LA)	Alpha-Linolenic Acid (ALA)
— Enzymes	— Enzymes
Gamma-Linolenic Acid (GLA)	Eicosapentaenoic Acid (EPA)
Enzymes —	Enzymes
Dihomo-Gamma-Linolenic Acid (DGLA)	Prostaglandin Series 3 / Less Inflammatory Leukotrienes
Prostaglandin Series 1 / — Enzymes	
Arachidonic Acid	
Enzymes	
Prostaglandin Series 2 / Pro-Inflammatory Leukotrienes	

Table 2

FOODS HIGH IN OMEGA-3 FATS	FOODS HIGH IN OMEGA-6 FATS
• Cold-water fish (salmon, mackerel, tuna, sardines, and herring)	• Black currant oil
• Flaxseeds and flaxseed oil	• Borage oil
• Perilla oil	• Grape-seed oil
• Walnuts and walnut oil	• Sesame oil
• Purslane	• Evening primrose oil
• Wheat germ oil	• Walnuts and walnut oil
	• Corn oil
	• Safflower oil
	• Sunflower seeds and sunflower seed oil
	• Cottonseed oil
	• Soybean oil
	• Hempseed oil
	• Brazil nuts
	• Margarine
	• Pumpkin and squash seeds
	• Spanish peanuts
	• Peanut butter
	• Almonds
	• Wheat germ oil

essary for normal growth, hair and skin health, regulation of metabolism, and reproduction. Omega-3 fatty acids, along with omega-6 fatty acids, are now considered essential fats that must be included in your diet. The major sources of omega fats are listed in Table 2.

There is also an omega-9 fatty acid called oleic acid, a monounsaturated fat found most notably in olive oil. It has a range of talents, particularly in cardiovascular health and cancer protection, although it is not an essential fat. You'll learn more about all of these beneficial fats throughout this book.

Listed in Table 3 are the various types of dietary fat and their sources, functions, and recommended intake.

Other Forms of Fat

In addition to triglycerides, two other types of lipids are the sterols (which include cholesterol) and phospholipids. Cholesterol is an odorless, waxy, fatlike substance found in all foods of animal origin. It is a chemical cousin of fat. Needed for good health, cholesterol is a constituent of most body tissues and is used to make certain hormones, vitamin D, and bile, a substance involved in the digestion and absorption of fats. You'll learn more about cholesterol in the next chapter.

Phospholipids contain a molecule of phosphorus, which makes them soluble in water. This characteristic helps fats travel in and out of the lipid-rich membranes of cells. In fact, both cholesterol and phospholipids form part of the structure of cell membranes. A well-known phospholipid is lecithin, manufactured by your liver and found in many foods.

WHAT HAPPENS TO THE FAT YOU EAT?

When you feast on fat or fat-containing foods, it begins its digestion in your mouth, where special enzymes act on its breakdown. Fat then travels to your stomach, separates from other food components, and floats to the top of the stomach. Little fat digestion takes place here, however, since fat doesn't mix well with the watery fluids in your stomach.

Table 3

THE SKINNY ON FATS

Dietary Fats	Sources	Function	Recommended Intake
Saturated fat	Red meat, dairy products, coconut oil, palm oil, egg yolks	Provides energy, stimulates the liver to manufacture cholesterol	7 to 10 percent of total calories
Polyunsaturated fat	Corn, soybean, sesame, safflower oils; some fish	Provides energy, stimulates less bad cholesterol and more good cholesterol	Up to 10 percent of total calories
Monounsaturated fat	Olive, canola, peanut oils; avocado, some fish	Provides energy, stimulates less bad cholesterol and more good cholesterol	Up to 15 percent of total calories
Omega-3 fatty acids	Fish, including salmon, tuna, sardines, bluefish, trout; flaxseed oil	Polyunsaturated fats that reduce the risk of abnormal blood clotting; may help prevent heart disease	Increase as part of total recommended intake of polyunsaturated fats. Optimal ratio of omega-3 fats to omega-6 fats is 1:1; 1:4 is also considered healthy

Table 3 continued

THE SKINNY ON FATS

Dietary Fats	Sources	Function	Recommended Intake
Omega-6 fatty acids	Many vegetable oils, seeds, nuts, whole grains, fast foods, baked goods	Polyunsaturated fats that are involved in cellular health	Optimal ratio of omega-3 fats to omega-6 fats is 1:1; 1:4 is also considered healthy
Trans-fatty acids	Stick margarine, shortening, baked goods, fast foods, snack foods	Polyunsaturated fats that have been processed; they act like saturated fats in the body and are damaging to health	Limit or avoid

Fat next enters your small intestine. To assist with digestion here, your gallbladder squirts bile into your intestine at mealtimes. In a process called emulsification, a molecule of bile attaches itself to a molecule of fat, dispersing the fat into the watery solution where it can meet fat-splitting enzymes. Almost the same thing happens when you wash clothes. The detergent acts as an emulsifier to dissolve the grease, molecule by molecule, suspending it in water so that it can be rinsed away. Long-chain fatty acids require bile for digestion; short- and medium-chain acids do not.

If you've had your gallbladder removed, you can still digest fats. That's because the gallbladder only *stores* bile.

Bile is produced by your liver and delivered continuously into your small intestine, not just at meals. You'll be instructed to reduce your fat intake, however, because your body can handle only a small amount of fat at a time.

Enzymes split the triglycerides from their glycerol backbones, liberating the fatty acids, which then cross the membrane of the intestine where they are resynthesized back into fats. Some newly re-formed fats are so large that they must be wrapped in special protein blankets to get to their destinations. These protein blankets are called lipoproteins. Some lipoproteins carry a large amount of cholesterol. Elevated concentrations of these lipoproteins can be an early warning sign of heart disease.

Lipoproteins are picked up by the lymphatic system, a secondary circulatory system. It features an elaborate network of organs, tissues, and vessels whose major functions are to transport digested fat from the intestine to the bloodstream and to defend the body against invasion by disease-causing agents.

From the lymphatic system, lipoproteins are carried to the liver (the primary site of metabolism) for further processing. From there, the fat is released into the bloodstream, where it is picked up by fat cells and eventually stored as body fat, if not used immediately for energy. But because the body prefers to use glucose (blood sugar) first for fuel, fats (specifically longer-chain fats) tend to be stored as body fat. By contrast, short-chain fatty acids bypass the lymphatic system and are absorbed directly through a special vein that leads to the liver, where, inside the cells, they are rapidly oxidized or burned up. As you can tell, many complex reactions are involved in the digestion and absorption of dietary fats.

FAT—WHO NEEDS IT?

You do! Despite its bad rap, fat is a highly useful nutri-
ent, vital for life. As noted earlier, dietary fat provides
essential fatty acids, which are vitaminlike substances that
have a protective effect on your body. And once digested,
dietary fats help transport and distribute fat-soluble vitamins (vitamins A, D, E, and K) throughout your body so
that they can be stored in your liver and fatty tissue until
needed. Both dietary fat and stored fat have other important roles in the body:

Growth and Development

Fat—particularly the omega-3 fats—is needed for good
health throughout the life span, beginning in the womb.
A deficiency of omega-3 fatty acids during pregnancy can
affect a baby's growth and development, particularly mental and visual functioning. Children require essential fats
too, to support good health during their growth years.

A Source of Energy

Fat is a fuel that provides a substantial portion of energy
required to drive the body's basal metabolism, which represents the energy it takes just to exist—or, put another
way, the energy needed to control vital internal functions
such as breathing, heartbeat, hormone secretion, and the
activity of the nervous system. When needed, stored body
fat can be converted into an emergency energy supply to
help us stay alive in the event of a long famine, or during
a debilitating illness to provide energy to battle the disease.

Dietary fat is a highly concentrated source of energy.

One gram of fat provides twice as much energy (calories) as one gram of carbohydrate or protein. So if you're hiking or hunting, particularly in cold weather, you need lots of food energy to sustain yourself—food energy that's best supplied mostly by fat-rich foods.

Fat is considered an exercise fuel, but more of a second-string source of energy. During exercise, your body prefers to burn carbohydrate for energy, as glucose in your blood or glycogen stored in your muscles. But if carbohydrate dwindles, your body draws on fatty acids for fuel. In contrast to your limited but ready-to-use glycogen stores, fat stores are practically unlimited. In fact, it has been estimated that the average adult man carries enough fat (about a gallon) to ride a bike from Chicago to Los Angeles, a distance of roughly 2,000 miles.

Flavor Enhancement

Although fairly tasteless itself, fat imparts enticing flavor and aroma to foods, thus stimulating your appetite. You experience this every time you smell bacon frying or enjoy a spoonful of ice cream. What's more, cooking with fat makes meats and baked foods more tender, moist, and flavorful. If the cookies you ate for dessert "melted in your mouth," you have fat to thank for the sensation.

Appetite Control

Although fats stimulate your appetite, they can suppress it too. That's because fats are slow to digest and thus make you feel full after you've eaten a meal. They also stimulate the intestinal wall to secrete a satiety-control hormone called cholecystokinin (CCK), which acts on nerves in your stomach and slows the rate of digestion.

CCK is also released by the hypothalamus, the body's appetite control center. The net effect of CCK's release in the body is to tell the brain you're full. Worth mentioning too: Among fats, polyunsaturated fatty acids are more powerful than either saturated fats or monounsaturated fats in bringing on a feeling of fullness.

Fat Storage

Many dietary triglycerides (the food fat you eat) are shuttled to fat depots—in muscles, breasts, thighs, hips, the area under your skin, and other places—where they are stored. This occurs only after your body has used all the fats and carbohydrates it needs for energy.

Your body stores dietary fat much more readily than it does carbohydrates, which must first be dismantled into tiny fragments and reassembled into fatty acids—a complex process that requires lots of energy. But because dietary fat is so chemically similar to body fat, it requires fewer breakdown steps before it is stored. Therefore, if you eat the same number of excess calories from fat and carbohydrate, your body will store the fat calories rather than the carbohydrate calories. The more fat you eat, the more you're likely to wear.

It is this storage fat that we're always trying to get rid of. When you put on fat weight, storage fat cells—which are specialized for hoarding fat—become stuffed with fat and enlarge as a result. If you gain fifty pounds or more, fat cells start to multiply, and you've got them for life. Dieting doesn't obliterate fat cells either. It only shrinks them.

Protection and Insulation

But even storage fat serves some useful purposes. Some storage fat pads organs for protection and acts as a shock absorber, cushioning them from jolts. Most storage fat is found just under the skin, where it insulates us from extremes in temperature.

Storage fat makes up most of the 20 to 30 billion fat cells in our bodies. A smaller percentage of body fat—around 15 percent—is classified as "essential fat." It is the structural constituent of vital body parts such as the brain, nerve tissue, bone marrow, heart, and cell membranes. Storage fat is constructed from the essential fatty acids you obtain from your diet.

Hormone Production and Control

Fats are also required for hormone production and regulation. Produced by glands, tissues, and organs, hormones are chemical messengers that control various conditions in the body. While most hormones are secreted by glands, some are produced in fatty tissue. A good example is a lipid called 7-dehydrocholesterol, found in the fat just beneath the surface of your skin. It is activated by sunlight and converted into vitamin D, which has a number of hormonal duties in the body.

Fatty tissue is also involved in regulating the production of female sex hormones, mainly estrogen. Estrogen is the collective name for a trio of female hormones: estradiol, secreted from the ovaries during the reproductive years; estriol, produced by the placenta during pregnancy; and estrone, secreted by the ovaries and adrenal glands and found in women after menopause. These naturally occurring estrogens are responsible for developing the female sex characteristics, regulating menstrual cycles, and maintaining normal cholesterol levels.

At puberty, after a young girl has gained a certain percentage of body fat, she begins to menstruate and develop sexually. Throughout life, too much fat or too little fat can interfere with the ability to have normal periods, ovulate, and become fertile. Losing a lot of weight and depleting body stores, for example, leads to an estrogen deficiency similar to menopause, and periods cease.

A HEALTH-ENHANCING NUTRIENT

So you see: Fat is a valuable nutrient in your diet. And what's more, some fats are absolutely vital for good health. Without them, you're putting your well-being on the line.

As with any nutrient, the misuse of fat—whether from eating too much of it or not eating enough of certain kinds of fat—can detract from your health. In the next chapter, we'll take a look at this issue and delve into why some fats can be fatal.

TWO

When Fat Can Be Fatal

The reason fat has gotten such a bum rap has to do with America's number one killer—cardiovascular disease. Each day in the United States, cardiovascular disease claims more than 2,600 lives—an average of one death every thirty-three seconds, according to the most recent statistics from the American Heart Association.

The accepted explanation for such high rates of cardiovascular disease has been this: Saturated fats and cholesterol in our diets lead to high cholesterol in the blood, which in turn clogs blood vessels, contributing to heart attack and stroke. So for nearly forty years, we've been told that by shunning foods such as butter, cream, cheese, eggs, and meat—sources of saturated fats and cholesterol—and replacing them with low-fat, cholesterol-free foods, we can cut our risk of cardiovascular disease.

But there is a little bit more to the story. Emerging from decades of research is the fact that multiple factors appear to play a role in the development of cardiovascular disease: smoking, lack of exercise, high blood pressure, excess sugar consumption, poor diet quality—and fat. Thus, the fat/disease controversy is far from resolved. One thing is certain, though: The typical American diet is too high in certain types of fats with known links to disease. In this chapter, we'll look into the fat factor in disease—and why some fats promote illness and poor health.

SATURATED FAT, CHOLESTEROL, AND CARDIOVASCULAR HEALTH

Over time, too much saturated fat in your diet can harm the health of your cardiovascular system. Essentially, excess saturated fat disrupts your liver's ability to break down excess cholesterol, a fat that is a building block for cells and hormones. Further, saturated fat causes your liver to churn out cholesterol to form an artery-clogging type of cholesterol known as low-density lipoprotein (LDL) cholesterol, dubbed the "bad" cholesterol.

For background, cholesterol comes as cholesterol in your blood and cholesterol in food. Because your body can manufacture cholesterol from fats, carbohydrates, or proteins, you don't require cholesterol from food.

When you eat a food that contains cholesterol, that cholesterol is simply broken into smaller components of various fats and proteins that are used to make many other substances that your body requires. In other words, the cholesterol you eat doesn't raise the cholesterol in your blood. It's just that some foods high in cholesterol also happen to be loaded with saturated fat. The more saturated fat you eat, the more cholesterol your liver makes.

If your liver overproduces cholesterol and pumps out LDL cholesterol, the excess circulating in the bloodstream forms lesions inside the walls of your arteries, where it is eventually deposited. LDL cholesterol is highly susceptible to oxidation, a tissue-damaging process that occurs when oxygen reacts with fat—in this case, the lipid portion of LDL cholesterol. Oxidation is thought to play a role in the formation of these arterial lesions. Your body begins forming plaque as a biological bandage to repair the lesions. Trouble starts, though, when plaque builds up in an artery, narrowing the passageway and choking off blood flow. A heart attack can occur when blood flow to the heart muscle is cut off for a long period of time, and part of the heart muscle begins to die.

A body-friendly cholesterol is high-density lipoprotein, (HDL) cholesterol. It contains the least cholesterol and does not cause lesions. Its job is to pick up the bad cholesterol from the cells in the artery walls and transport it back to the liver for reprocessing or excretion from the body as waste. HDL cholesterol has been nicknamed the "good" cholesterol.

A medical test called the *blood lipid profile* detects the amount of cholesterol in your blood, which is considered a prime forecaster of your likelihood of suffering a heart attack or stroke. But it is not the only forecaster; others are smoking and high blood pressure (hypertension).

A total cholesterol reading above 200 may be a danger sign. Generally, HDL cholesterol should be higher than 35, while LDL should be 100 or below. Borderline high LDL is considered 130 to 159; high LDL, 160; and very high LDL, 190, according to new recommendations from the National Heart, Lung, and Blood Institute. High blood LDL cholesterol is therefore a major risk factor for heart disease, but one that can be controlled by losing weight, eating less saturated fat, and exercising more.

Some people, however, have high cholesterol no matter how well they watch their diets or exercise. That's because their livers are genetically programmed to over-produce cholesterol. In such cases and in certain high-risk cases, doctors may prescribe cholesterol-lowering drugs. Most work by interfering with a liver enzyme's ability to manufacture cholesterol.

When checking cholesterol, your doctor may be on the lookout for the *lipid triad,* which also increases your risk of cardiovascular disease. Essentially, the lipid triad describes the presence of elevated triglycerides (dietary fats not fully broken down by the liver that circulate in the blood), too-low HDL cholesterol, and high LDL cholesterol—in particular, a type of LDL cholesterol characterized by its small particle size. "Small" LDL cholesterol can get into artery walls more easily and cause damage more quickly than larger LDL particles can.

Interestingly, the lipid triad worsens not by eating a high-fat diet, but by indulging in a high-carbohydrate diet, especially one that is laced with refined carbohydrates and sugary foods. Although it reduces LDL cholesterol, a high-carbohydrate diet lowers the good HDL cholesterol and elevates your triglycerides. Here's why: If you load up on carbohydrates—without burning them up—your liver will convert them into saturated fat. So eating lots of carbohydrates, even though you're forfeiting fat, doesn't do your heart much good.

SATURATED FAT AND CANCER

Diets high in saturated fat have been linked to certain types of cancers, largely because animal studies beginning in the 1950s began to show evidence of an association. However, this link is not an open-and-shut case. Take breast cancer, for example—the most extensively studied cancer in terms of its relationship to dietary fat.

Until fairly recently, saturated fat was believed to be a criminal in the promotion of breast cancer. However, a study of nearly 90,000 women conducted by doctors at Boston's Brigham and Women's Hospital exonerated saturated fat, finding little evidence of the suspected breast cancer link. Other research has produced similar findings. Most investigators believe that multiple factors are at work to increase the risk of breast cancer—including genetics, menstrual history, sedentary lifestyle, body fat, and overall diet—so it's difficult to pin the cause on saturated fat alone.

Diets overloaded with saturated fats have also been implicated in the development of prostate cancer and colon cancer. With regard to prostate cancer, saturated fat is thought to alter levels of sex hormones, an environment that can promote cancer. In a study recently conducted in France, investigators found that men whose diets contained more than 30 to 40 percent fat (most of it saturated) had a higher risk of developing prostate cancer than men whose diets contained less than 30 percent fat.

The risk of colon cancer catching up with you sometime in the future may be related to the amount and type of fat you eat. A Harvard study discovered that men who ate low amounts of saturated fat (7 percent of their calories) had half the rate of precancerous polyps than men who ate double that amount (14 percent). Polyps can progress into tumors in the colon.

As for the type of fat you eat, oil from fish has been found to protect against colon cancer, in contrast to the possible cancer-promoting effect of saturated fat. What's more, in countries where people consume a lot of olive oil, rates of colon cancer are very low.

Keep in mind that the link between saturated fat and

cancer is still under debate in scientific circles. Rather than point fingers at saturated fat only, scientists and nutritionists have begun to emphasize the importance of overall dietary quality, specifically the need to eat more vegetables, fruits, whole grains, fiber, and other nutrient-packed foods, in order to reduce your cancer risk.

Saturated Fat and Inflammation

Saturated fats promote the production of arachidonic acid, the fatty acid that gives rise to inflammatory agents in the body, namely bad prostaglandins (series 2) and pro-inflammatory leukotrienes. These agents can harm your joints, leading to arthritis, and can trigger abnormal blood clotting and thus promote clogged arteries. Bad prostaglandins and leukotrienes have also been implicated in migraine headaches and psoriasis. By reducing the amount of saturated fat you eat, it's quite possible to tame the production of inflammatory substances in your body.

THE UGLIEST OF ALL: HYDROGENATED AND TRANS-FATTY ACIDS

In truth, the real culprit in life-threatening diseases may turn out not to be saturated fat, but a super-deadly fat known as *hydrogenated* or *partially hydrogenated* fat. Examples include margarine and vegetable shortening. Hydrogenated fats are also used in commercially baked products, including cakes, doughnuts, cookies, crackers, potato chips, and other snack foods.

Hydrogenated fats are polyunsaturated omega-6 fatty acids that have been synthetically altered in a process called hydrogenation. To produce them, manufacturers take the cheapest oils available—usually soy, corn, or cottonseed—which are already rancid from the extraction process, then bubble hydrogen into the oil. Nickel oxide, which is quite toxic, is also used in the process, and traces are left in the final product. In the case of margarine, other chemicals are added (most notably bleach and coal-tar dyes) to make it look like butter.

Hydrogenation changes the chemical makeup of the fat to harden it, make it more spreadable than the original oil, and keep it fresh longer. But consequently, the unsaturated fatty acids become saturated as they take on the hydrogen and behave more like saturated fats in your body. The original fat is robbed of its unsaturated properties and healthful benefits.

There's more: During hydrogenation, some of the unsaturated fats, rather than turning into saturated fats, change their shape and morph into unnatural fats called trans-fatty acids. These fats are loathsome to your body. They slink into cell membranes, making them rigid, inflexible, and generally impaired. Consequently, the victimized cells are handicapped, unable to protect themselves against invaders or circulate freely through blood vessels.

Some major research into the effects of trans-fatty acids on health reveals the rather threatening nature of these fats. A landmark Harvard study found that women who ate four or more teaspoons of margarine a day had a 66 percent higher chance of heart disease than women who ate less than one teaspoon a month. The probable cause: Trans-fatty acids inhibit the body's ability to properly use essential fatty acids (the good fats) and elevate cholesterol.

The cholesterol-elevating problem associated with trans-fatty acids was revealed in a study conducted in the

Netherlands. Investigators observed that trans-fatty acids raised levels of LDL cholesterol to the same degree that saturated fats did. And according to another study, cooking with margarine is health-risky, increasing your odds of heart disease by 90 percent. The Framingham Heart Study, a long-term study monitoring the health status of 5,127 men and women from Framingham, Massachusetts, also found that eating margarine increased the risk of heart and artery disease.

Diets overloaded with trans-fatty acids may increase your risk of breast cancer too. That's the finding of a University of North Carolina study showing that women whose fatty tissue contained high levels of trans-fatty acids and low levels of essential fatty acids were three times more likely to develop breast cancer.

Other research has found that diets high in hydrogenated and trans-fatty acids are linked to other serious problems: prostate cancer, diabetes, obesity, immune disorders, low-birth-weight babies, lactation problems, sterility, and bone disorders. Without a doubt, you should stay away from these bad fats. Here are some guidelines for steering clear of hydrogenated and trans-fatty acids:

- Read food labels. Even foods claiming to be cholesterol-free, low-fat, or natural may contain trans-fatty acids. That being so, avoid food products that have the words *hydrogenated* or *partially hydrogenated* on their labels.

- Limit or avoid using stick margarine, which is the most highly hydrogenated fat of all. Softer tub and liquid margarines are lower in trans-fatty acids, and are a better alternative. In fact, a study conducted at the University of Texas Southwestern Medical Center revealed that tub margarine reduced LDL cholesterol by an average of 10 percent in adults and children over a five-week period.

+ Butter isn't necessary a bad choice if you're a spread lover. That's because it contains no trans-fatty acids. Just use a dab, though, since butter is high in saturated fats. (See Table 4 for important information on butter.)

+ Avoid cooking with stick margarine or shortening. Substitute vegetable oil. Or, for a fat-free recipe, replace the fat with applesauce or fruit purée.

+ Choose margarines and other fats that contain liquid vegetable oil as the first ingredient and no more than two grams of saturated fat per tablespoon.

+ Cut back on foods that are fried in vegetable shortening, such as French fries or fried chicken.

+ Use olive oil in place of margarine for dipping breads, rolls, or bagels.

+ Use olive oil or canola oil to sauté vegetables and other foods.

+ Check out the new margarines made without trans-fatty acids. These include trans-free olive oil spreads; spreads made with a blend of soy, canola, olive, and palm oils; and trans-free, fat-free margarines and spreads (these use carbohydrate-based fat replacers rather than fat).

Table 4

THE CASE FOR BUTTER

Butter is not the bad guy it's been made out to be. Consider the following facts:

- The idea that butter elevates cholesterol has not been well substantiated by research. Margarine is a worse offender.
- Butter is a good source of fat-soluble vitamins such as vitamins A, D, and E. In fact, vitamin A from butter is more readily absorbed than from other sources.
- Chemically, butter consists of short- and medium-chain fatty acids, which are absorbed directly from the small intestine to the liver for quick energy and less of a tendency to be stored as body fat.
- Butter contains lauric acid, the only saturated fatty acid not made by the body. Lauric acid is notable because it fights disease-causing microorganisms and tumors, and it helps bolster the immune system. In excess, however, lauric acid increases cholesterol levels in the blood.
- Butter contains two very-short-chain fatty acids—proprionic acid and butyric acid—that have antifungal and antitumor powers.
- Butter is rich in selenium, an antioxidant mineral.
- A natural constituent of butter is lecithin, a phospholipid involved in the proper metabolism of cholesterol.

THE TRUTH ABOUT TROPICAL OILS

Cast as fat villains on the nutritional stage are a group of saturated fats known as the tropical oils. They include coconut, palm, and palm kernel oils, and the cocoa butter in chocolate. Tropical oils are generally found in commercial baked goods and other processed foods because they impart an appealing flavor and consistency to these foods and extend their shelf life.

Coconut oil, for example, is added to some nondairy creamers and nondairy dessert toppings to replace butterfat (cream). But ironically, coconut oil is more saturated than cream. It has been shown in studies to raise cholesterol levels and is thus likely to increase the risk of heart disease. Palm kernel oil elevates cholesterol too and is considered risky, as well.

Palm oil, on the other hand, is much less of a villain. Though saturated, palm oil elevates the good HDL cholesterol, prevents abnormal clotting in the blood, and reduces blood pressure. Plus, it contains vitamin E, an important antioxidant that helps keep cholesterol in check. Another healthful component of palm oil is oleic acid, a monounsaturated fatty acid plentiful in olives and olive oil. Oleic acid has beneficial effects on cholesterol levels.

As for cocoa butter—the fat found naturally in chocolate—the news is good. Studies show that it does not adversely affect heart health the way many other saturated fats do. There's more: A Harvard study found that men who ate chocolate one to three times a month lived longer than men who ate none.

Does this mean chocolate is a health food?

Not exactly. However, cocoa butter is rich in a saturated fatty acid called stearic acid, also found in meat and dairy products. Research shows that stearic acid does not elevate cholesterol, nor does it promote heart attacks. Further, it prevents the formation of dangerous blood clots.

This encouraging information isn't a license to go overboard on chocolate, however. Scientists and nutritionists advise that chocolate can still be savored, but in moderation, since it is high in calories and fat.

When it comes to tropical oils, there are villain fats (coconut oil and palm kernel oils) and hero fats (palm oil and cocoa butter). Many food manufacturers, however, have removed tropical oils from cookies, cakes, and crackers. A word of caution, though: Some of these fats, particularly coconut and palm oils, will show up as hydrogenated or partially hydrogenated fats in various food products. Read labels, and try to avoid these types of fats.

WHEN POLYUNSATURATED FATS GO BAD

Generally, when saturated fats are replaced in the diet with polyunsaturated fats—specifically those of the omega-3 and omega-6 families—cholesterol levels drop. But the problem is that polyunsaturated fats, particularly the omega-6 fatty acids, cut all cholesterol—the bad kind (LDL) and the good kind (HDL). Omega-6 fats are found in commercial vegetable oils made from corn, soy, safflower, sunflower seeds, and peanuts. To make matters worse, cancer researchers have discovered a close correlation between diets high in omega-6 fatty acids and a greater risk of cancer.

But aren't polyunsaturated fats supposed to be good for you?

Yes—they are among the healthier fats. But a problem with polyunsaturated fats is that they are highly vulnerable to oxidation, a process in which fat is exposed to oxygen and turns rancid as a result. As polyunsaturated fats sop up oxygen, they can be attacked by free radicals and converted into harmful molecules called *lipid peroxides*. Peroxides attack cell membranes, setting off a chain reaction that creates many more free radicals. Pits form in cell membranes, allowing harmful bacteria, viruses, and other disease-causing agents to gain entry into cells. Other structures such as body proteins, DNA (the genetic material inside cells), and cartilage can be attacked by free radicals and damaged too. The result is a frenzy of cell destruction. Lipid peroxidation is believed to be one of the mechanisms involved in the development of autoimmune diseases, heart disease, and cancer.

Food processing encourages oxidation. Thus, foods most likely to contain rancid, oxidized polyunsaturated fats are processed food products—crackers, snack foods, frozen foods, cookies, pastries, baked goods, and packaged foods, among others.

Always read the labels of processed foods. Shun them if the label lists polyunsaturated fats such as safflower oil, sunflower seed oil, corn oil, soybean oil, or peanut oil, because you can bet they are oxidized. Opt for fat-free foods instead.

Another problem, specifically with omega-6 fats, is that in excess they stimulate the formation of arachidonic acid, which is a precursor or building block of "bad" prostaglandins and pro-inflammatory leukotrienes that are involved in inflammation. Although we need some arachidonic acid, too much is believed to be responsible for the rise in arthritis and other chronic inflammatory diseases. An oversupply of arachidonic acid also fuels the growth of cancer cells.

RISKY BUSINESS: LOW-FAT DIETS

If you're a Jack Sprat—that is, you eat little or no fat— you risk an essential fat deficiency, which can be as health-damaging as eating too much of the wrong kind of fat. Case in point: A study published in the medical journal *Metabolism* found that in forty-seven patients with heart disease, blood levels of essential fatty acids were significantly lower than levels found in healthy people. Ouch!

Further, a study in the *British Journal of Nutrition* showed that a low-fat diet can affect your mood—in a bad way. In this study, ten men and ten women ate a higher-fat diet (41 percent of calories from fat) for one month, then switched to a low-fat diet (25 percent of calories from fat). While on the higher-fat diet, volunteers experienced less tension and anxiety, suggesting that cutting fat may make you feel down in the dumps. The study didn't specify why this may have occurred, but it is well known that essential fats promote good mental functioning.

Some scientists feel that essential fatty acid deficiency may be the most serious dietary health problem facing Americans. With fat-slashing diets, the body has trouble absorbing the fat-soluble vitamins A, D, E, and K. Furthermore, the health of cell membranes is jeopardized because low-fat diets are low in vitamin E. Vitamin E is an antioxidant that prevents disease-causing free radicals from puncturing cell membranes.

So valuable are essential fatty acids that deficiencies can cause a wide range of serious symptoms and illnesses. Table 5 lists the physical conditions that can be brought on by a short supply of essential fatty acids. Clearly, you'll want to make sure your diet provides ample essential fats for good health.

PUTTING BAD FATS IN PERSPECTIVE: A DISEASE-PREVENTION STRATEGY

Saturated fats and other bad fats should not receive all the blame for heart disease and other life-shortening ill-

Table 5

ESSENTIAL FATTY ACID DEFICIENCY:
SYMPTOMS AND ILLNESSES

Fatigue	Arthritis
Dry skin and hair	Chest pain
Cracked nails	Cardiovascular disease
Dry mucous membranes (mouth, tear ducts, vagina)	High blood pressure
Digestive problems	Memory problems
Constipation	Depression
Poor immunity	
Frequent colds	
Joint problems	

nesses. Few pieces of evidence bring this so clearly into focus than a landmark study published in the *New England Journal of Medicine* in 2000. For fourteen years, Harvard researchers followed more than 84,000 women participating in the Nurses' Health Study. They were free of heart disease, cancer, and diabetes in 1980—when the study began. By the end of the study, women at the lowest risk of disease, particularly heart disease, were those who did not smoke and exercised at least a half hour daily. Further, they followed diets that were high in fiber, folic acid (a B-vitamin that protects against heart disease), and good fats (those from fish and vegetables), and were low in trans-fatty acids and sugar.

Translation: It's the totality of your lifestyle, not just one unhealthy portion of it, that most affects your disease risk. That being the case, here's what you can do to stay as healthy as you can, for as long as you can:

Reduce your intake of saturated fats and trans-fatty acids in favor of unsaturated fats. According to the American Heart Association, the maximum amount of fat considered healthy in your daily diet is 30 percent or less, based on the number of calories you eat over several days, such as a week. To translate this recommendation into meaningful terms, a 2,000-calorie diet should contain about sixty-five grams of fat a day.

Saturated fat and trans-fatty acids combined should be 7 to 10 percent or less of total daily calories; polyunsaturated fats should also be at 10 percent or less; and mono-unsaturated fats should make up to 15 percent of total calories. Dietary cholesterol should be kept to a daily maximum of 300 milligrams or less (200 milligrams or less if you suffer from high cholesterol).

Quit smoking. Each year, smoking kills approximately 500,000 Americans. Heart attack, lung cancer, and chronic lung disease are the chief smoking-related diseases that claim human life. Yet death from smoking doesn't have to happen. It is the single largest preventable cause of premature death and disability.

Maintain a normal weight for your height and body frame. After smoking, weight-related conditions are the second leading cause of death in the United States, claiming 300,000 lives each year. Although overweight and obesity are considered to be appearance problems, they are in fact serious conditions, directly linked to a number of disabling and life-threatening diseases. Among them: coronary heart disease, stroke, some cancers, diabetes, high blood pressure, gallbladder disease, osteoarthritis, and mental health problems. The best way to determine a normal weight is to have your body fat percentage tested. Generally, a body fat percentage between 18 and 24 percent for women and between 15 and 18 percent for men is considered optimal.

Exercise at a moderate-to-vigorous pace for at least thirty minutes most days of the week. An estimated 250,000 deaths in the United States each year are linked to a lack of exercise, according to the Centers for Disease Control and Prevention. It's well established by research that exercise protects you against heart disease, cancer, obesity, bone diseases, and many other life-limiting illnesses.

Fill up with fiber. Most plant foods, including cereals, pasta, fruits, and vegetables, are complex carbohydrates that are packed with dietary fiber, an indigestible carbohydrate that has a long list of impressive health benefits. Fiber has a cholesterol-lowering effect, and it helps relieve constipation, rid the body of cancer-causing substances, and assist in weight control. The National Research Council recommends 20 to 35 grams of fiber a day.

Eat fish two to three times a week. Fish contains beneficial fats that are endowed with numerous health benefits. You'll learn more about the health-boosting powers of fish and fish oils in chapter 3.

Obtain enough folic acid. Found in green leafy vegetables, this B-vitamin reduces homocysteine, a proteinlike substance, in the tissues and blood. High homocysteine levels have been linked to heart disease. Scientists predict that as many as 50,000 premature deaths a year from heart disease could be prevented by increasing consumption of folic acid.

Recent scientific experiments have revealed that folic acid deficiencies cause DNA damage that resembles the DNA damage in cancer cells. This finding has led scientists to suggest a link between cancer and a folic acid deficiency. Other studies show that low levels of folic acid

appear to be associated with premalignant cell growth in
the cervix. The recommended daily intakes of folic acid
are as follows: women, 400 micrograms; pregnant
women, 600 micrograms; lactating women, 500 micrograms; and men, 400 micrograms.

Reduce your intake of refined carbohydrates. These
foods include sugar, sweets, breads, and processed snack
foods. Such foods provoke metabolic problems that promote fat storage, elevate blood fats, and raise blood pressure. Sugar, in particular, lowers your body's resistance
to disease and creates deficiencies in heart-protective B-
vitamins.

PART II

Omega Healing

THREE

Fishing for Good Health

Question: What do heart disease, arthritis, cancer, diabetes, bowel disease, psoriasis, and depression have in common?

Answer: All of these troubling ills can be treated effectively with a group of essential polyunsaturated fats called omega-3 fatty acids. Omega-3 fatty acids come in three varieties: alpha-linolenic acid (ALA), eicosapentaenoic acid (EPA), and docosahexaenoic acid (DHA).

Alpha-linolenic acid, which must be obtained from your diet, is found mostly in plant foods such as flax, soybeans, and vegetables. From these foods, it is converted to EPA and DHA in your body. EPA and DHA are also found in fish, where they are *preformed*. This simply means that they don't require conversion from alpha-linolenic acid and thus are better utilized by the body. You can thus obtain EPA and DHA directly from fish and shellfish.

Seafood is the richest source of EPA and DHA in our food supply. Cold-water fish such as salmon, mackerel, and tuna supply the most EPA and DHA because they swim around in chilly waters and develop a thick layer of insulating fat to keep warm. If not for the abundant un-saturated fatty acids in these fish, their fat would solidify in the cold-water environment, and the fish would be un-able to swim.

In addition, cold-water fish feed on plankton, which contains alpha-linolenic acid (the original aquatic source of EPA and DHA) and algae, which is chock-full of DHA. But if you're not a fish eater, don't worry. You can obtain EPA and DHA from dietary supplements. Table 6 pro-vides information on the amount of omega-3 fatty acids found in various food sources and supplements.

HEALING POWER FROM FISH

For more than twenty-five years, research reports have been pouring in over the potent health benefits of omega-3 fatty acids. Their healthful properties first came to light when scientists discovered that Greenland Eskimos have a lower rate of heart disease and stroke than other popu-lations do, despite their high-fat diet. The difference is that Eskimos eat twenty times more fish than Americans, and fish is loaded with omega-3 fatty acids.

Because of this link, omega-3 fatty acids have become best known for their good deeds in cardiovascular health, where they have been found to lower blood pressure, re-duce cholesterol, thwart dangerous blood clotting, and protect against irregular heartbeats.

Basically, your body uses omega-3 fats to manufacture eicosanoids (prostaglandins and leukotrienes), hormone-like substances that regulate many chemical processes. As noted in chapter 1, prostaglandins come in two varieties:

Table 6

OMEGA-3 FATTY ACID CONTENT OF FOODS

	Food (per 100 grams)	ALA (grams)	EPA + DHA (grams)
Oils	Perilla oil	63.6	0
	Flaxseed oil	53.3	0
	Black currant oil	12–14	0
	Canola oil	11.1	0
	Soybean oil	6.8	0
Nuts and Seeds	Walnuts, English	6.8	0
	Walnuts, black	3.3	0
	Soybean kernels	1.5	0
Vegetables	Soybeans, green, raw	3.2	0
	Soybean sprouts	2.1	0
	Purslane	0.4	0
	Beans (navy, pinto)	0.3	0
Fish	Sardines, in sardine oil	0.5	3.3
	Atlantic mackerel	0.3	2.5
	Atlantic salmon	0.1	1.8
	Pacific herring	0.1	1.7
	Atlantic herring	0.1	1.6
	Lake trout	0.4	1.6
	Bluefin tuna	trace	1.6
	Anchovy	trace	1.4
	Atlantic bluefish	trace	1.2
	Pink salmon	trace	1.0
	Bass, striped	trace	0.8
	Florida pompano	trace	0.6
	Halibut, Pacific	trace	0.4
	Catfish	trace	0.3
	Cod	trace	0.3
	Flounder	trace	0.2
	Haddock	trace	0.2
	Red snapper	trace	0.2
	Swordfish	trace	0.2

Table 6 continued

OMEGA-3 FATTY ACID CONTENT OF FOODS

	Food (per 100 grams)	ALA (grams)	EPA + DHA (grams)
Shellfish	Alaska king crab	trace	0.3
	Shrimp	trace	0.3
	Lobster	trace	0.2
Mollusks	Oyster	trace	0.6
	Mussel, blue	trace	0.5
	Scallop	trace	0.2
	Clam	trace	trace
Supplements	Promega		44.2
	MaxEPA		29.4
	Salmon oil		19.9
	Cod liver oil		18.5

Adapted from: Nettle, J.A. 1991. Omega-3 fatty acids: comparison of plant and seafood sources. *Journal of the American Dietetic Association* 91: 331–337; Connor, W.E., et al. 1993. (N-3 fatty acids from fish. *Annals of the New York Academy of Sciences* 14: 16–34.)

the good prostaglandins, which have healing properties, and the bad prostaglandins, which promote disease and inflammation. Likewise, there are less inflammatory leukotrienes and pro-inflammatory leukotrienes. An imbalance of fat in the diet—namely, too much saturated fat and omega-6 fatty acids—promotes the production of bad prostaglandins and leukotrienes.

By contrast, increasing omega-3 fatty acids through diet steps up the production of good prostaglandins and less inflammatory leukotrienes in the body. As a result, omega-3 fats can alter your metabolism in four positive ways: They slow the rate at which your liver manufactures triglycerides; they make your blood less sticky, so that clots are less likely to form; they help repair tissues that have been damaged by lack of oxygen (a condition that occurs when arteries become blocked and can't deliver oxygen to the heart or brain); and they help lower blood pressure, a risk factor for heart attacks and stroke. In addition, omega-3 fats act like white knights of sorts, protecting the body when its own immune system attacks tissues, as in rheumatoid arthritis.

Thus, omega-3 fats have been heralded for their ability to treat an amazing array of other diseases, from heart disease to cancer. Here's a closer look.

Battle Heart Blockages

Elevated levels of cholesterol and triglycerides are risk factors for heart disease. In excess amounts, cholesterol can collect in the inner lining of the arteries and lead to a heart attack. Triglycerides are a type of fat that circulates in your blood. When levels are too high, HDL cholesterol (the good kind) tends to fall. Omega-3 fats have been found to influence both cholesterol and triglycerides. A few examples:

In one study, patients who supplemented with three tablespoons of fish oil every day reduced their total cholesterol by 15 percent in just four weeks. One specific type of fish oil—salmon oil—reduces triglycerides, cholesterol, and a harmful type of cholesterol known as VLDL (very-low-density lipoprotein) in people with an excess of blood fats in their system. Salmon oil has also been found to increase HDL cholesterol, the beneficial kind.

But in other cases, fish oil has performed poorly as a cholesterol-lowering agent. A Mayo Clinic statistical study, called a meta-analysis, of about twenty-one trials involving people with type 2 diabetes found that while fish oil (ranging from 3 to 18 grams daily) slashed triglyceride levels, it unfortunately raised levels of harmful

LDL cholesterol, particularly in individuals who used the higher doses. Other studies have found that fish oil has very little effect on cholesterol except when patients have elevated triglycerides.

On a more positive note, some experiments have discovered that fish oil can abort or prevent the formation of lesions in the walls of your arteries. Caused by oxidized LDL cholesterol, these lesions make it possible for cholesterol to collect in the arteries and eventually plug them up. Fish oil thus protects your arteries from damage and saves them from potential blockages.

It's vital to note that eating fish rich in omega-3 fats, rather than taking fish oil supplements, may be a better prescription for keeping your arteries healthy. Canadian researchers found that people who ate more than eight ounces of fish a week stood a better chance of having their arteries stay open after angioplasty (a procedure that dilates arteries) than patients who ate no fish. Another study showed that taking fish oil capsules did not keep arteries open following angioplasty.

Regulate Normal Blood Clotting

There are two chemicals in your body that, in the right balance, are responsible for preventing abnormal blood clots but assuring the prompt formation of clots when you're cut or bruised, in order to control bleeding and help you heal. These chemicals are thromboxane and prostacyclin.

Thromboxane, a prostaglandin mainly synthesized from arachidonic acid, is the chemical that tells platelets—tiny clotting factors in your blood—to clump together, forming blood clots. But should one of these clots wend its way into a blood vessel narrowed by atherosclerosis (hardening and thickening of the arteries), it could trigger a heart attack or stroke. Prostacyclin, synthesized mostly from EPA, orders platelets to not stick together and move along.

If a platelet has too much arachidonic acid in its cell walls, more thromboxane is produced, and the platelet will clot too easily, possibly leading to heart attack or stroke. By contrast, if a platelet has enough EPA in its cell wall, less thromboxane is made, prostacyclin becomes more potent, and blood stays more fluid.

Supplying your body with ample amounts of omega-3 fats keeps thromboxane and prostacyclin production in proper balance. Consequently, dangerous clots are less likely to form.

Heal Hypertension

Known as the silent killer, high blood pressure (hypertension) afflicts about 60 million Americans, half of whom do not know they have it. Hypertension is a serious condition because it contributes to heart attacks and strokes. Blood pressure exceeding 140/90 spells danger and should be brought under control. Prescriptions for high blood pressure include exercising, restricting salt intake, cutting down on alcohol and caffeine, quitting smoking, losing body fat, and taking blood pressure medication.

To that list, we can add consuming fish and fish oil— and justifiably so. Taking 3,000 milligrams of fish oil (the amount in seven ounces of fatty fish) a day reduces high blood pressure, according to a meta-analysis of seventeen controlled clinical trials of the effect of fish oil supplements on high blood pressure.

In another study, volunteers ate a mackerel diet containing about 5 grams of omega-3 fats every day. Their blood pressure fell moderately, from 152/93 to 140/89, on average. With slightly more omega-3s (6 grams daily),

blood pressure may drop even lower, from 147/82 to 124/
74, according to other research.

It's not clear exactly how fish and fish oil reduce blood
pressure, but scientists theorize that the same chemicals—
thromboxane and prostacyclin—that help control blood
clotting are believed to lower blood pressure. Thromboxane constricts blood vessels, while prostacyclin dilates
them. When in balance, these chemicals help arteries relax
and stay flexible, causing a reduction in blood pressure.

Protect Against Irregular Heartbeats

Each year in the United States, about 300,000 people die
within one hour of suffering a heart attack, primarily due
to irregular heartbeats (arrhythmias) stemming from damage to heart tissue. Arrhythmias occur when the electrical
system that controls your heartbeat is disturbed. The ven-
tricles, the lower chambers of your heart, begin to contract
rapidly and chaotically, resulting in insufficient blood flow
to your vital organs.

Evidence is mounting that a simple dietary change—
eating more omega-3 fats—may help prevent fatal arrhythmias. Research with isolated cardiac cells of rats
shows that omega-3 fats enhance the electrical stability of
heart cells. Specifically, omega-3s help regulate the or-
derly flow of calcium, sodium, and other charged particles
into heart cells to ensure normal contractions.

In a study involving human volunteers, people took 4.3
grams of a fish oil supplement every day for sixteen
weeks. At the end of the study, the fish oil–takers had a
marked reduction in the average number of arrhythmias—
from 5.9 to 2.9.

Eating fish also helps keep the heart from beating ir-
regularly. Case in point: 295 men who ate just one fatty-

fish meal a week had half the risk of heart failure due to arrhythmia.

No one can yet guarantee that fish or fish oil will fully prevent arrhythmias, but if you want to hedge your bets, eat more fish or consider supplementing with fish oil.

Relieve Arthritis

One of the most promising uses of fish and fish oil has been in the treatment of rheumatoid arthritis, a joint disease in which the body's own immune system attacks its tissues. More than 2 million people have this form of arthritis. Most are women.

The chief symptoms of rheumatoid arthritis are pain, swelling, and stiffness—all thought to be triggered by pro-inflammatory prostaglandins called leukotrienes, which are synthesized from arachidonic acid. In a rather dramatic nutritional rescue, omega-3 fatty acids interfere with the conversion of arachidonic acid to leukotrienes, thus reducing their levels in the body and rendering them less inflammatory.

In a study conducted at Albany Medical College, sixty-six rheumatoid arthritis patients were given either fish oil supplements (130 milligrams per kilogram of body weight) or nine capsules of corn oil, every day for thirty weeks. All patients continued to take their regular prescription medicine during the study. As the study progressed, joint tenderness and morning stiffness decreased significantly in patients taking fish oil supplements. Some of the patients were able to stop taking their prescription medicine due to the pain-relieving effects of fish oil supplements.

This study is just one of the many trials that have been conducted, showing such encouraging results. Generally, fish oil provides moderate relief from symptoms and makes patients less reliant on anti-inflammatory drugs and pain medication. The effective dose for arthritis relief appears to be 3 to 5 grams of omega-3 fatty acids a day. That's the equivalent of eating about 8 ounces of omega-3-rich fish every day.

If you want to cut your chances of developing rheumatoid arthritis, you can get by with less—1.6 grams of omega-3 fatty acids per day or two or more servings of fish per week, according to recent studies.

Here's more good news for your joints: Omega-3 fatty acids may protect you against a more prevalent form of arthritis called osteoarthritis (a joint disease in which cartilage gradually deteriorates). Again, the proof comes from Eskimos, who have the lowest rates of osteoarthritis in the world. As noted earlier, they eat a diet rich in fish oils, namely omega-3 fatty acids, which appear to have a protective effect on joints. But in Eskimos who become "westernized," the rate of osteoarthritis triples.

Another beneficial source of joint-soothing omega-3 fatty acids is the green-lipped mussel, a dietary staple of people living in coastal areas of New Zealand. Not coincidentally, these New Zealanders have very low rates of arthritis compared to their inland neighbors, and scientists have long believed that the mussel is the reason. For nearly thirty years, extracts made from the green-lipped mussel have been a popular curative for arthritis in New Zealand and Australia.

One of these extracts is Lyprinol, a supplement derived from the green-lipped mussel that has been fairly well researched as an anti-inflammatory treatment for various diseases, including arthritis. Studies indicate that Lyprinol (210 milligrams daily) relieves symptoms associated with rheumatoid arthritis and osteoarthritis, with few side effects. It appears to work by interfering with the synthesis of a troublesome inflammatory leukotriene called B4, making it less inflammatory.

Fight Cancer

The cancer-fighting potential of omega-3 fatty acids has been studied for nearly twenty years, mostly in lab animals. Still, the findings have been exciting, particularly in the ability of omega-3s to suppress tumor growth. A large body of animal studies shows that omega-3 fats slow the growth and spread of tumors, prolong survival, and even prevent tumors from forming.

Fish and fish oil may powerfully thwart breast cancer too, according to population studies of large groups of people living in various regions of the world. Scientists have found that rates of breast cancer are lowest in Japan and other countries where women eat the most fish.

Scientists theorize that omega-3 fatty acids work by countering the harmful effects of bad prostaglandins, which lower immunity and promote cancer growth. When levels of these not-so-friendly prostaglandins are too high, the body can't protect itself and tumors tend to grow faster.

As research into the antitumor activity of omega-3s continues, it will be fascinating to see how it all shakes out. But until more information is available, it does seem a wise idea to eat more seafood on a regular basis.

Counter the Complications of Diabetes

The value of fish and fish oil in treating diabetes, a blood-sugar-metabolism disorder, is in countering the life-threatening complications of the disease. One of these is heart disease, the leading cause of death in people who suffer from diabetes. In fact, the death toll among diabetics with heart disease is about two to four times as high as those adults without diabetes. One reason is that people with diabetes often have high levels of blood lipids (cholesterol and triglycerides) and thus are at greater risk of developing atherosclerosis.

Fish oil has the most profound effect on lowering triglycerides—often dropping by as much as 30 percent. Conducted in the Netherlands, a statistical study of twenty-six clinical trials involving diabetics discovered that fish oil doses (ranging from 1.8 to 20 grams daily) slashed triglyceride levels, but generally had little effect on LDL or HDL cholesterol. The researchers suggested that if you have diabetes, there's room for fish oil supplements in treating triglycerides that are on the high side, particularly if standard therapies fail.

Ease Bowel Disease

In addition to heart disease and osteoarthritis, there's something else Eskimos rarely get: inflammatory bowel disease (specifically Crohn's disease and ulcerative colitis). Crohn's disease is painful, chronic inflammation of the intestine, and though rare, it seems to be on the rise. Ulcerative colitis is also a chronic condition, characterized by tiny ulcers in the inner lining of the colon.

Quite a few studies show that omega-3 fatty acids provide relief from both conditions. They work primarily by reducing the levels of that rather nasty leukotriene called B4, which is elevated in the gastrointestinal tracts of people with inflammatory bowel disease. If you have either of these diseases, try eating more fish or taking fish oil supplements, while adhering to your regular medical treatment.

Treat Psoriasis

Affecting approximately 3 million Americans, psoriasis is a genetic disease in which the life cycle of skin cells fast-forwards abnormally, and the result is skin eruptions and scaling. Psoriasis typically affects the elbows, knees, trunk, and scalp. Conventional treatment involves medications and phototherapy (exposure of the skin to ultraviolet light). But research suggests that fish oil, particularly eicosapentaenoic acid (EPA), is also an effective way to manage the disease.

People with psoriasis have higher-than-normal amounts of inflammatory leukotrienes, namely B4, in their bodies. These are believed to trigger the characteristic inflammation and scaly skin of this disease. In one study, twenty-eight psoriasis patients each were given 1.8 grams of EPA, or an olive oil placebo, every day for two months. By the end of the experimental period, itching and redness were reduced in people taking the EPA supplement. Other research indicates that EPA supplements taken with etretinate (a drug that treats psoriasis) work better than the drug by itself. If you're under the care of a doctor for psoriasis, it might be worth adding fish oil supplements to your treatment to get some relief from the itching and inflammation.

Defeat Depression

Depression, a mental illness that affects one of every four Americans, is a very common mental disorder. In fact, it has been dubbed "the common cold" of psychiatric problems—but it is the most treatable, provided the sufferer seeks treatment.

One form of treatment now getting a lot of attention in scientific circles is supplementation with omega-3 fatty acids. By studying the differences between people who get depressed and those who don't—a type of research known as psychiatric epidemiology—scientists first discovered the fascinating link between omega-3 fats and mood. Epidemiological studies have found that countries with the highest rate of fish consumption—most notably New Zealand and Japan—have very low rates of depression. Because of this knowledge, doctors and mental health experts are now suggesting that we eat more fish for protection against depression. One type of omega-3 fat—DHA—is particularly effective for escaping depression. You'll learn more about this important fatty acid in the next chapter.

A landmark study conducted at Harvard suggested that fish oil supplements (6 grams daily) can relieve symptoms of manic depression, also known as bipolar disorder, a form of depression characterized by unpredictable mood swings.

Scientists also believe that one of the instigators of postpartum depression—the down-in-the-dumps feeling experienced by some mothers a few days after delivery—is the depletion of maternal omega-3 fatty acids, a common nutritional deficiency during pregnancy. In a study of fish consumption in twenty-seven countries and the development of postpartum depression, researchers found that the more fish women ate, the less they experienced this form of depression.

Exactly how omega-3 fats help alleviate mood disorders such as depression and bipolar disorder is a puzzle. But there are some clues. Some studies suggest that higher

levels of essential fatty acids in plasma may lead to increased levels of neurotransmitters—brain chemicals that
transmit messages from one nerve cell to another—particularly serotonin. Serotonin is known as the "happiness
neurotransmitter" because elevated levels bring on feel-
ings of tranquillity, calm, and emotional well-being. Low
levels may increase the risk for depression.

Another theory holds that the inflammatory response
runs amok in people with mood disorders, and as a result,
the body starts cranking out too many disease-fighting
substances. When in excess, these substances hurt normal
cell function and reduce levels of serotonin and other neurotransmitters. But because of their ability to thwart inflammation, omega-3 fatty acids may put the brakes on
out-of-control inflammatory processes.

Other Benefits

In addition to protection against disease and depression,
omega-3 fatty acids may boost your performance if you're
an exerciser. In a study of thirty-two healthy men, researchers found that supplementation with omega-3 fatty
acids boosted aerobic power almost as much as aerobic
exercise itself.

Also, omega-3 fatty acids have the ability to dilate the
capillaries. This improves the flow of oxygen and nutrients muscles during exercise and facilitates the removal
of waste products. The more nutrients the muscles can
get, the better the conditions are for growth and repair.

Because of their role in the production of good prostaglandins, omega-3 fatty acids may also reduce exercise-
caused inflammation and allow your muscles to repair
faster following exercise.

THE PROMISE OF SHARK LIVER OIL

For more than forty years, one specific type of fish oil—
shark liver oil—has been used medicinally as an alternative treatment for various diseases, including cancer. Its
most familiar use, however, is as an ingredient in topical
hemorrhoid creams. Shark liver oil is also available in
supplements sold in health food stores.

A longtime popular therapeutic agent in Europe, shark
liver oil is a major natural source of two beneficial compounds—squalene (see chapter 7 on olive oil) and alkylglycerols. Alkylglycerols are a group of lipids similar in
structure to triglycerides. Found in fatty fish, as well as
in human bone marrow and breast milk, alkylglycerols
have been scientifically studied since the 1930s for their
ability to reduce radiation damage, suppress tumor
growth, build blood, and accelerate wound healing.

More recently, they have been researched for their role
in stimulating the immune system by empowering a type
of immune cell called a *macrophage*. Macrophages are
"search and destroy" cells on the lookout for foreign invaders, particularly bacteria and tumor cells. Before macrophages go out on their search-and-destroy mission, they
must be activated by other immune cells. It's a rather
complicated process, but once activated, macrophages can
secrete some sixty substances designed to kill disease-
causing agents. Scientists have discovered that alkylglycerols are capable of activating macrophages too. This
discovery has prompted research into alkylglycerols as antitumor compounds.

In various studies, alkylglycerols do appear to be useful
partners in cancer treatment. For example, when breast
cancer cells were treated in lab dishes with chemotherapy
or with chemotherapy and alkylglycerols, the combination

treatment reduced tumor cells in eight out of nine patient samples. In another study, alkylglycerols inhibited tumor growth and tissue damage after radiation in women undergoing treatment for cervical cancer. Experiments have also found that patients with uterine cancer who were treated with alkylglycerols prior to radiation treatment lived longer and had a higher rate of tumor regression.

The effectiveness of alkylglycerols in reducing radiation damage may have to do with their antioxidant power, scientists believe. Although a useful therapy, radiation sets in motion a process in which the body begins spewing out devilish free radicals called *hydroxy radicals*, capable of attacking whatever they contact. Hydroxy radicals have been implicated in numerous diseases, as well as in aging. Research suggests that alkylglycerols inhibit the formation of these cellular renegades, or neutralize them at the moment of their genesis.

Numerous supplement companies manufacture shark liver oil capsules. The usual dosages are capsules with 250 to 500 milligrams of shark liver oil containing 20 percent alkylglycerols (50 to 100 milligrams of alkylglycerols). For supportive therapy during conventional cancer treatment or for immune-deficient diseases, medical experts familiar with shark liver oil recommend taking three to six 500-milligram capsules daily; for immune support and disease prevention, two to three 250-milligram capsules daily. Be sure to get your physician's blessing before supplementing, however.

OMEGA-3 HEALING POWER FROM PLANTS

As noted earlier in this chapter, alpha-linolenic acid is an omega-3 fat found mostly in plants and seed oils.

Alpha-linolenic acid is a *precursor*, or building block, of EPA and DHA. However, nutritionists will tell you that it is better to get EPA and DHA directly from fish because they are better absorbed and utilized by your body.

Even so, there are health benefits to eating vegetables high in alpha-linolenic acid, since it affords significant protection against heart disease, stroke, and other illnesses. Foods rich in alpha-linolenic acid include flaxseed and perilla oil. You'll learn more about these important foods in chapter 5.

THE ALL-IMPORTANT OMEGA RATIO

Historically, our ancestors ate higher amounts of omega-3 fatty acids than we do today. In fact, our intake of omega-3 fats is pitifully low—which is why rates of heart disease, cancer, and other dreaded diseases may be escalating. The blame for the shift in omega-3 fat consumption can be placed mostly on food processing, which has dumped dangerous trans-fats into our foods through the process of hydrogenation. We're also eating too many omega-6 fatty acids from vegetable oils. That's bad because excess omega-6 fats interfere with the conversion of alpha-linolenic acid to EPA and DHA, and they spur the production of bad prostaglandins and leukotrienes. Our overindulgence in saturated fats has also displaced omega-3 fats in our diets.

Currently, we eat about 12 grams of omega-6 fats a day to 1.5 grams of omega-3 fats. This fat imbalance has led many nutrition and medical experts to recommend increasing omega-3 fats in our diets to achieve a more balanced ratio between omega-3 fats and omega-6 fats. Some authorities have suggested a 1:1 ratio, which would put as much omega-3 fats in our cells as omega-6 fats. This is the ratio found in the traditional diet of Greece, where deaths due to heart disease and cancer are among the lowest in world. Even by cutting our omega-6 intake in half and doubling our omega-3 intake, we'd achieve a more healthy balance.

How can we restore the balance?

There's really no magic dietary formula. Simply change your present diet to include more seafood and vegetables, while cutting back on processed foods and saturated fats, and you'll automatically balance the ratio in favor of omega-3 fats in your diet.

EATING MORE FISH

Generally, the best way to harness the healing power of omega-3 fats is to eat more seafood. Here are some guidelines:

- Eat two to three three-ounce fish meals a week to decrease your odds of heart disease, cancer, arthritis, and other illnesses. Just a four-ounce portion of salmon twice a week, for example, serves up about 5 grams of omega-3 fatty acids, the amount recommended by most health care practitioners.

- Not all types of fish supply the same amount of omega-3 fats. It's best to choose fattier fish such as salmon, tuna, mackerel, or sardines most of the time, since they contain the most omega-3 fats.

- Substitute fish for red meat. Research shows that this practice can alter your cholesterol profiles for the better.

- Prepare fish by broiling, grilling, microwaving, baking, or poaching. Frying can be self-defeating because the fish is often cooked in not-so-healthy oils.

- Shellfish is not off-limits if you have high cholesterol. Research shows that shellfish, which contains cholesterol, has a minimal effect on cholesterol levels. So for variety, don't be afraid to enjoy crab, oysters, shrimp, scallops, and other shellfish.

SOME FISHY PRECAUTIONS

Some species of fish may be contaminated with toxins, so if you eat too much of them to get your omega-3 fats, you might be ingesting too many chemicals and pollutants. Some examples of fish that may be high in toxins include grouper, marlin, orange roughy, swordfish, and shark. According to the FDA, these species have tested for high levels of mercury (considered a poison) and should be eaten no more than twice a week, or, if you're pregnant, no more than once a month.

To be on the safe side:

- When purchasing fish, select a smaller fish within the species. It is typically younger and probably hasn't been exposed to toxins for as long as older, larger fish have.

- Buy farm-raised fish, if available. These are raised under controlled conditions, with less exposure to toxins and bacteria.

- Don't eat the skin or fatty portion of fish, because this is where toxins tend to congregate.

* Avoid eating the same species of fish all the time, to minimize possible exposure to the pollutants over and over again. In other words, plan your diet to include a variety of fish.

USING FISH OIL SUPPLEMENTS

Most doctors and medical researchers suggest that you eat more seafood—at least two to three fish meals a week—rather than rely on fish oil supplements. But if you don't like fish, supplements may be a good option. Some words to the wise if you choose this alternative:

* Supplementing with 3 grams of fish oil daily from food sources and/or dietary supplements is considered a safe dose by the Food and Drug Administration (FDA). But taking more than 3 grams daily may thin your blood and prevent it from clotting normally. Higher doses should be taken only under medical supervision.

* Fish oil supplements are not without other side effects. An excess of these oils can be harmful and cause internal or external bleeding. Other side effects include belching, gas, nausea, heartburn, diarrhea, and fish odor on your breath or from your body.

* Take fish oil supplements with your meals to help minimize fishy breath and heartburn.

* Being a fat, fish oil supplements are high in calories and dietary cholesterol. A single capsule or softgel, for example, contains roughly 15 calories; some recommended dosages (multiple capsules daily) supply 200 extra calories a day. Unless you figure this into your

total daily caloric intake, you could pack on unwanted pounds. As for cholesterol, one study found that supplements can contain as much as 600 milligrams of cholesterol per 100 grams.

- Do not supplement if you're pregnant or lactating, since high doses of fish oil may affect the health of your child.

- Do not take cod liver oil as a source of omega-3s; it is high in vitamin A and vitamin D, which in large amounts can be toxic.

- Fish oil supplements may increase your requirement for vitamin E, so ask your doctor if you would benefit from taking vitamin E supplements.

- Avoid fish oil supplements if you're taking blood-thinning medications (including aspirin), since the combination may increase your risk of bleeding.

- Avoid taking fish oil supplements two weeks before and one week after surgery, because these supplements can interfere with blood clotting.

- Some fish oil supplements may contain pesticides or other toxic contaminants.

- Discuss with your physician the advisability of taking fish oil supplements, especially if you are under medical care for a serious illness.

FOUR

DHA:
The Brain-Building Fat

Though derogatory, the term fat head *is a rather apt* description of the brain. Fat makes up about 60 percent of your gray matter, and about a third of that fat is an omega-3 fatty acid called docosahexaenoic acid (DHA). There's even more DHA—50 to 60 percent—in the retina, a thin membrane attached to the back of your eye that senses and processes light images projected through your eyes.

Considered a building block of the brain, DHA is required for normal brain and eye development, as well as for mental well-being and visual functioning. In fact, your brain cells take up DHA in preference to other fatty acids.

DHA is also a constituent of cell membranes. One of its primary jobs is to protect the fluidity of brain cell membranes to ensure the normal transmission of nerve signals.

DHA is the most abundant omega-3 fatty acid in breast milk. Moreover, it is also found naturally in fish. No wonder, then, that fish is called a "brain food." Red meat, eggs, flaxseed, and certain vegetable oils contain appreciable amounts too.

Deficiencies of DHA are linked to numerous health problems, including atherosclerosis, autoimmune diseases, arthritis, cancer, mental disorders, cancer, metabolic disorders, and nervous system problems.

DHA has been intensely researched in recent years and the findings are quite impressive. DHA has the following positive effects:

Banishes Bad Moods

Low levels of DHA are linked to depression, a mental illness that affects one of every four Americans. Case in point: A study published in the medical journal *Lancet* stated that in regions where people ate more fish, there were fewer cases of depression. What's more, researchers reported in the *American Journal of Clinical Nutrition* noted that the documented increase in depression in North America in the last century parallels the dwindling consumption of DHA over the same period.

In other research, scientists have examined the cell membranes of people suffering from depression to assess cellular DHA levels. One study of fifteen depressed patients and fifteen healthy volunteers found that the depressed patients had significant depletions of essential fatty acids, particularly DHA, in the cell membranes of red blood cells. Considering the evidence, many mental health experts are advocating DHA supplements as a natural treatment for mild to moderate depression.

Rejuvenates Your Brain

Some researchers speculate that DHA, because of its importance in human brain tissue, may help prevent degenerative brain diseases such as dementia, memory loss, and Alzheimer's disease. In fact, a study conducted at Tufts University discovered that a low level of DHA is a significant risk factor for these brain diseases. One reason for the shortfall may be due to the body's decreasing ability to synthesize DHA as we age. Another possible explanation, say scientists, is inadequate nutrition among the elderly. Research is now being conducted to learn whether supplementation with DHA can avert age-related declines in mental function.

Enhances Memory

DHA may bring about memory improvement, according to an animal study conducted at Shimane Medical University in Japan. Using rats bred on a fish oil–deficient diet, investigators fed DHA to one group of animals and a placebo to another for ten weeks. The goal of the study was to learn whether DHA supplementation would have any effect on two types of memory: *reference memory*, which is information you learn and retain to perform a task the next time around; and *working memory*, another term for short-term memory.

DHA enhanced reference memory, but not short-term memory. The evidence: DHA-supplemented rats made fewer mistakes while negotiating a maze than the placebo-fed rats did.

Moreover, examination of the rats' brains revealed a possible biological clue for the improved memory: increased DHA in both the hippocampus, a sea horse–

shaped structure deep within the brain that helps you learn and remember; and the cerebral cortex, an area of the brain associated with visual memory and recollection. Based on these observations, the investigators suggested that DHA levels in the brain may indeed influence learning ability.

Treats Attention-Deficit Hyperactivity Disorder (ADHD)

Some preliminary evidence indicates that less-than-adequate levels of DHA are correlated with behavioral problems in children. A Purdue University study found significantly lower levels of DHA in children with attention-deficit hyperactivity disorder (ADHD), compared to controls. Generally affecting children, ADHD is the habitual inability to pay attention for more than a few moments and is accompanied by erratic activity.

Boosts Kids' Brainpower

Children who were breastfed as infants generally have higher intelligence and greater academic achievement than infants who were formula-fed, according to studies spanning more than twenty years. Consider: One study found that breastfed babies have a 38 percent greater likelihood of completing their high school education than formula-fed babies.

Some researchers speculate that DHA, which is found naturally in breast milk, may be one of the reasons for the better-than-average mental functioning in children who were breastfed as newborns. Studies do show that breastfed infants have higher levels of DHA in their brains than do formula-fed babies, so there may be some connection.

Unlike in European and Asian countries, infant formula

in the United States is not enriched with DHA, so the only way babies can get this vital fatty acid is through breast milk. Unfortunately, though, breast milk levels of DHA in American moms are among the lowest in the world. For comparison, the DHA in the breast milk of Europeans is double that of American women, and the breast milk of Japanese women is three times as rich in DHA. Breast milk is considered the best source of DHA for infants.

Thus, in the United States, many health care practitioners recommend eating more fish if you're pregnant or lactating. Another natural food source of DHA is flaxseed oil. You can also take a daily DHA capsule, but consult your physician first.

Saves Your Infant's Sight—and Yours

Not only is DHA vital for an infant's brain development, it is also essential for normal visual development and healthy eyesight. As noted earlier, DHA accounts for more than a third of the fatty acids in the retina and strengthens brain cells associated with eyesight. In a mother's womb, DHA is taken up preferentially by the placenta and travels directly to the unborn baby's brain and retinal tissue. During the final months of pregnancy and within the first six months of infancy, the retina undergoes rapid development, drawing upon stored energy and large amounts of DHA for growth.

If an expectant mother's body is DHA-needy or her newborn does not get enough DHA during these critical stages of retinal development, the child's visual health may be compromised. Evidence for this comes from a couple of studies. In a study published in the *American Journal of Clinical Nutrition*, children who were breastfed for four months had better stereoscopic vision at age three and a half than children who were not breastfed. Stereoscopic vision is the ability to see objects in three dimensions. What's more, children whose mothers ate oily fish during their pregnancies had better stereoscopic vision than those whose mothers who avoided fish.

Similarly, a study from the Retina Foundation in Dallas, Texas, discovered that newborns fed formula without DHA for a year had poorer vision than babies fed breast milk.

Does DHA confer a vision-protecting effect in adults too? Scientists think so. In a study reported in the *Archives of Ophthalmology,* investigators found that people who ate more fish, which is rich in DHA, had fewer incidences of age-related macular degeneration, the leading cause of legal blindness in the United States.

Treats Schizophrenia

Another potential use of DHA lies in treating schizophrenia, a destructive distortion of thinking in which a person's interpretation of reality is severely abnormal. Substantial evidence shows that chemical abnormalities in the brain cause schizophrenia.

A growing number of researchers are convinced that one of these abnormalities may be caused by low levels of DHA in brain cells and in red blood cells. British psychiatric researchers discovered that the depletion of essential fats, including DHA and arachidonic acid, is triggered largely by free-radical attacks on the membranes of red blood cells in patients with schizophrenia.

Boosting dietary levels of DHA may help, they found. After eating more essential fatty acids, including DHA, patients with schizophrenia had fewer symptoms after just six weeks.

Some startling research has revealed that newborns deprived of breast milk may be at risk of developing schizophrenia later in life. In a 1997 study published in the *British Journal of Psychiatry,* investigators suggest that a lack of brain-building DHA may contribute to this risk. They found that patients who were not breastfed had more schizophrenic traits and were more poorly adjusted than their breastfed siblings.

Protects the Heart

Enriching the diet with DHA lowers triglyceride levels by 26 percent, increases the good HDL cholesterol by 9 percent, and elevates apoprotein-E (a compound that ferries cholesterol from tissue back to the liver for breakdown and excretion) by 69 percent, according to a four-month study conducted by the U.S. Agricultural Research Service (ARS). That's encouraging news, particularly if you're trying to get your blood lipids under control.

Compared to fish oil supplements, isolated DHA seems to outperform on a number of fronts. For one thing, DHA does not result in such side effects as increased bleeding time or slower-than-normal blood clotting, both of which can occur with fish oil supplementation. Taking fish oil supplements also seems to elevate bad LDL cholesterol; taking DHA supplements does not.

Lowers Blood Pressure

Supplementing with DHA may help you defeat rising blood pressure. In a study conducted at the University of Western Australia, fifty-six men (ages twenty to sixty-

five) took 4 grams of either DHA, EPA, or an olive oil
placebo every day for six weeks. All the men were overweight, which is a risk factor for high blood pressure.
Among the lipids, DHA was the only one that had any
significant effect, lowering systolic pressure (upper number) by 3.5 points and diastolic pressure (bottom number)
by 2 points during the day. The benefits were modest, but
the researchers speculated that DHA may be the fatty acid
in fish most responsible for regulating blood pressure.

Controls Blood Sugar

Research with lab animals hints that supplementing with
DHA may put the brakes on a condition called *insulin
resistance*. A hormone with multiple jobs in the body,
insulin is required to move blood sugar (glucose) into
cells for energy and nourishment. But in cases of faulty
sugar metabolism, cells don't respond to insulin properly.
Consequently, glucose is locked out of cells, and it clut-
ters up the bloodstream.

The pancreas (where insulin is made) is forced to pump
out more of the hormone to handle the excess glucose in
the blood. But eventually, the pancreas can't keep pace
with the demand, so there's a flood of both insulin and
glucose in the bloodstream. This situation is a ticking time
bomb that can explode into diabetes, and with diabetes,
the potential and gradual deterioration of organs and blood
vessels—unless blood sugar can be brought under control.

Researchers in Japan observed that DHA reduced glucose levels in DHA-supplemented mice—a finding they
attribute to DHA's ability to make cells less resistant to
insulin. In other words, DHA somehow altered cellular
metabolism, allowing insulin to perform its job of pushing
glucose into cells. Though far from conclusive, this study

presents some intriguing evidence in favor of a diabetes-fighting benefit of DHA.

SUPPLEMENTING WITH DHA

*You can increase your supply of DHA by eating more cold-*water fish (the current recommendation is two to three fish meals a week), incorporating a tablespoon a day of flax-seed oil into your diet, or taking DHA supplements. Also important: Limit or avoid excessive alcohol consumption, since chronic alcohol intoxication depletes DHA in brain cells.

Generally, DHA supplements are manufactured from fish oil. However, one product—Neuromins—is made from marine algae, the fish's original DHA source, through a special extraction process. This product is free of toxins that may be present in some fish oils.

The recommended dosage of DHA is 100 milligrams a day for healthy adults who obtain some DHA from fish and other sources. If you eat little or no fish, 200 milligrams a day is recommended.

DHA is a fatty acid that is naturally present in various foods, and so it is digested just like any other fat. It appears to be very safe, with virtually no known side effects. As with any dietary supplement, you should consult a health care professional before taking supplemental DHA.

FIVE

Nature's Disease Fighters

Two good fats that could upstage a headliner like fish oil are now—bit players called flaxseed oil and perilla oil. Both are highly concentrated sources of the omega-3 fat alpha-linolenic acid, which has a windfall of health benefits. If you started eating both of these oils on a regular basis, you'd probably escape such feared diseases as heart disease, stroke, cancer, and arthritis, to name just a few.

JUST THE FLAX, MA'AM!

For background, flaxseed oil comes from the crushed seeds of the flax plant, a blue flowering plant cultivated in Europe, South America, Asia, Canada, and parts of the United States. Historically, the flax plant has been used as medicine since at least 3000 B.C. Later, in 650 B.C., Hippocrates, "the Father of Medicine," prescribed flaxseed as a curative for intestinal problems. The eighth-century king Charlemagne issued laws governing and protecting the plant, so important was flaxseed for the health of his subjects.

Flaxseed is a widely recognized folk remedy throughout the world, and today many health-conscious consumers are eating it for its many healthful benefits. Flaxseed is officially approved by the German Commission E— Germany's version of our FDA—for treating constipation, diverticulitis, irritable bowel syndrome, and colons damaged by laxative abuse.

Worth mentioning too: On many farms, chickens are fed rations containing flaxseed so that they will lay omega-3-enriched eggs. In fact, these eggs contain eight to ten times more omega-3 fatty acids than regular eggs.

Though flaxseed is not a universal cure-all, this much is certain: Flaxseed and flaxseed oil display astonishing powers against many life-shortening diseases. This power emanates from the various constituents of flaxseed. Flaxseed oil is simply the world's richest treasure trove of omega-3 fatty acids. In fact, it has more than double the amount of omega-3s found in fish. So if you're not a fish eater, you can still get plenty of omega-3s by eating flaxseed and flaxseed oil.

Flaxseed is also a super source of alpha-linolenic acid (ALA), yielding 57 percent ALA—compared to 10 percent ALA found in the next-highest sources, canola and walnut oils. Flaxseed oil also contains 16 percent linoleic acid (an omega-6 fatty acid), 18 percent monounsaturated fatty acids, and only 9 percent saturated fatty acids.

Another ingredient in flaxseed worth knowing about is a group of beneficial phytochemicals (plant chemicals) called *lignans,* which work in monumentally important ways. First, they are thought to act as antioxidants, saving cells from destructive free radicals. Second, they also function as phytoestrogens, weak versions of estrogen found in fruits, vegetables, and whole grains.

Phytoestrogens are therapeutic in that they have a split personality. In premenopausal women, who have a lot of circulating estrogen, phytoestrogens cause the body to produce less of the hormone. Yet they work just the opposite way in postmenopausal women, who have low levels of the hormone, by increasing levels of estrogen. Many health practitioners believe that the estrogen-regulating effects of phytoestrogens may be helpful in fighting hormone-dependent cancers, such as breast or uterine cancers. Indeed, women who eat a lot of lignans have lower rates of breast cancer, according to research.

Lignans are found in numerous plant foods—namely barley, buckwheat, millet, oats, legumes, vegetables, and fruits—but nowhere are they as abundant as in flaxseed. Flaxseed boasts 75 to 800 times more lignans than any other food in the plant kingdom. Flaxseed oil, however, contains negligible amounts of lignans, which are nearly all removed during the oil-extraction process.

Flaxseed is loaded with fiber too, with about 6 grams in a fourth of a cup—more than twice as much as you'd get in a comparable serving of pure wheat bran. Research shows that adding flaxseed to your diet promotes regularity.

If you're really serious about enhancing your health, it's time to get serious about flaxseed. Here is a more detailed look at its health-giving properties.

Unclogs Arteries

Eating about 3½ tablespoons of milled flaxseed daily (in muffins) reduces artery-clogging LDL cholesterol by 18 percent and total cholesterol by 9 percent, a Canadian study found. Animal studies indicate that the lignans in flaxseed are responsible for the cholesterol-lowering effect.

Scientists believe that lignans, which are antioxidants, suppress the activity of free radicals before they have a chance to oxidize cholesterol and damage the interior linings of the arteries. Investigators at the University of Saskatchewan, who have conducted the bulk of this research, note that supplementing with flaxseed could "prevent hypercholesterolemia-related heart attack and strokes." Hypercholesterolemia is the medical term for high cholesterol.

Further, postmenopausal women who ate bread and muffins containing 38 grams of flaxseed flour lowered their total cholesterol from 229 to 213 and their LDL from 158 to 133, on average. Significantly, flaxseed reduced levels of a protein called *lipoprotein a,* which increases after menopause and contributes to the development of atherosclerosis, the narrowing and thickening of arteries that is responsible for heart attacks.

Prevents Second Heart Attacks

As stated earlier, flaxseed is loaded with alpha-linolenic acid (ALA). In a five-year study of survivors of a first heart attack, researchers found that those who followed an ALA-enriched diet, compared to those who followed a standard low-fat diet, had fewer second heart attacks over the experimental period. The researchers noted that the ALA-enriched diet appeared to be effective in preventing second heart attacks, but added that more research is needed to confirm a benefit.

Normalizes Clotting Function

In a twenty-three-day study involving college-age men, flaxseed oil (40 grams daily) exhibited "antiplatelet" activity. This means it prevents platelets from clumping together when they're not supposed to in an abnormal process called platelet aggregation. Platelet aggregation triggers the formation of dangerous blood clots called *thrombi* (singular, *thrombus*). A heart attack occurs when a thrombus obstructs a blood vessel supplying oxygen and nutrients to the heart muscle. The researchers concluded that alpha-linolenic-rich oils such as flaxseed may offer protection against cardiovascular disease complicated by the potential for blood clots.

Thwarts Cancer

Flaxseed displays cancer-fighting power, possibly due to its abundance of lignans. As noted, lignans are phytoestrogens that may protect against certain kinds of cancer, particularly hormone-dependent cancers such as those of the breast and prostate.

Studies at the University of Toronto showed that daily doses of flaxseed shrank mammary tumors in rats by more than 50 percent after seven weeks of treatment. Again, scientists believe that the tumor-reducing effect is due to lignans. So promising is the animal research that flaxseed is being tested to shrink breast tumors prior to surgery in women with breast cancer. Lignans have also been shown in animal studies to keep new tumors from sprouting.

Other animal studies show that flaxseed protects against colon cancer—a benefit that is also linked to lignans—and prevents the spread (metastasis) of this deadly cancer.

Boosts Immunity

The omega-3 fatty acids in flaxseed favorably affect your immune system by beefing up the content of alpha-linolenic acid, docosahexaenoic acid (DHA), and eicosapentaenoic acid (EPA) in the membranes of immune cells. Increasing the omega-3 content of cell membranes does two important duties. First, it helps encourage the formation of beneficial prostaglandins and leukotrienes. Second, it inhibits the formation of proteins that promote inflammation, encourage cancer, and interfere with normal cell function. One study showed that eating a flaxseed oil–enriched diet for eight weeks suppressed the production of these harmful proteins by 77 to 81 percent in a group of men. Bottom line: Flaxseed appears to inhibit harmful reactions leading to cell damage.

Prevents Diabetes

Diabetes is a sugar metabolism disorder in which the body does not produce any insulin (type 1 diabetes), or can't use it properly (type 2 diabetes). Some diabetes investigators believe that free-radical damage may contribute to diabetes by damaging insulin-producing cells in the pancreas. In type 1 diabetes, especially, cells in the pancreas are naturally low in levels of protective antioxidants that neutralize free radicals.

Now it appears that adding flaxseed to your diet may be a good defense against free-radical damage to the pancreas, according to a Canadian study. The study found that rats treated with a lignan isolated from flaxseed were protected from developing type 1 diabetes. According to investigators, the lignan shored up antioxidant defenses and prevented *oxidative stress*—a situation that occurs when protective antioxidants are swamped by destructive free radicals. Flaxseed oil may also boost blood circulation, which is often sluggish in people with diabetes.

FLAXSEED OIL VS. FISH OIL

There's no question that supplementation with fish oil confers some demonstrable health benefits, particularly in normalizing cholesterol and blood pressure. But so does flaxseed oil. The reason for their therapeutic power is that both oils are rich in omega-3 fatty acids. So the question is: Which oil is better if you want to acquire the healing power of omega-3 fatty acids?

Here are a few things to consider. Some fish oil supplements have been found to be adulterated with high levels of *lipid peroxides*. These harmful by-products form when free radicals hook up with fatty acids. Lipid peroxides attack cell membranes, setting off a chain reaction that creates many more free radicals. Pits form in cell membranes, allowing harmful bacteria, viruses, and other disease-causing agents to gain entry into cells. Thus, a better strategy may be to eat more fish and supplement your diet with flaxseed oil, rather than rely on fish oil supplements for your omega-3 fatty acids.

Further, flaxseed oil:

+ Has less tendency to turn rancid

+ Is not contaminated with toxic substances (fish oil supplements are rarely pure and often contain concentrations of highly toxic chemicals)

+ Is more economical (at recommended dosages, fish oil

can cost an average of $40 to $100 a month, while
flaxseed oil averages between $6 and $18 a month)

PURCHASING QUALITY FLAXSEED OIL

There are many manufacturing variations in the way flax-
seed oil is made from seeds, but generally it is produced
by mechanically extracting and pressing the oil through
an expeller press. The process generates a tremendous
amount of heat, which can easily damage the oil's essential fatty acids. The higher the temperature, the greater the
yield. Unfortunately, many manufacturers sacrifice quality
for quantity.

Because of the variations in processing, not all flaxseed
oil has the same quality. Nor does it possess the same
therapeutic potential. Thus, when shopping for flaxseed,
purchase the best-quality oil you can find. To help you,
here are some guidelines recommended by herbalists and
alternative health practitioners:

- Purchase flaxseed oil from a health food store. Generally, health food stores carry brands from quality
  manufacturers. In addition, make sure the oil is found
  in the refrigerated case of the store. Storage at room
  temperature for prolonged periods can degrade the po-
  tency of the oil.

- Check to see whether the oil is produced by *modified
  expeller presses* at temperatures that do not exceed 98
  degrees Fahrenheit. Some of the trade names to look
  for are Bio-Electron Process, Spectra-Vac, and Ome-
  gaflo. Do not purchase oil that has been *cold pressed.*
  This is a very deceiving term because processing tem-

peratures can reach 200 degrees Fahrenheit, even though no external source of heat is used.

* Make sure the product is packaged in an opaque (light-resistant) container. Contact with light can degrade the oil and destroy its healthful properties.

* Purchase an oil that is certified as organic by a third-party source. Stated on the label, certification ensures that the oil is free from pesticides and herbicides.

* Check the expiration date of the oil and adhere to these dates. You can freeze flaxseed oil, however, and thus extend its expiration date indefinitely.

USING FLAXSEEDS AND FLAXSEED OIL

The two best ways to get the benefits of flaxseed are to add whole flaxseeds or flaxseed oil to your diet. For good health, the recommended dosage is 1 tablespoon of whole seeds for every 100 pounds of body weight. You can sprinkle flaxseeds on your cereal in the morning—they have a delicious nutty flavor—put them in salads, mix them into yogurt or applesauce, or bake them into muffins and breads in place of nuts. The alpha-linolenic acid and lignans in flaxseeds remain stable when batters and doughs containing them are baked at customary baking temperatures.

You can also mill the seeds in a coffee grinder to yield a finer consistency. Ground seeds can be added to various recipes to enhance the flavor and nutrition of foods. Because of their rich oil content, ground seeds can replace all of the oil or shortening in recipes. If a recipe calls for one-third cup of oil, for example, use 1 cup of ground seeds instead (a 3-to-1 substitution). Also, one ½ cup of ground flaxseed can replace ½ cup of butter, margarine, or shortening. Baked goods using seeds in this manner will brown more rapidly.

You can also substitute ground flaxseed for eggs in recipes if you are a vegetarian or are cutting back on eggs. The substitution is as follows: 1 tablespoon ground flaxseed plus 3 tablespoons of water = 1 egg. Let the flaxseed/water mixture sit for 1 to 2 minutes before using in the recipe.

For treating gastrointestinal problems, *The PDR for Herbal Medicines* suggests taking 1 tablespoon of whole seeds with a half cup of liquid two to three times a day. Whole seeds should be stored in a cool, dry place and can be kept for one year. In addition, shop for flax-enriched foods, which are turning up in health food stores and some grocery stores.

Another option is to consume 1 tablespoon of flaxseed oil daily, in the form of a flaxseed salad dressing or mixed into food. Flaxseed oil is digested and absorbed better when eaten with food. Recipes for using flaxseeds and flaxseed oil are found in chapter 12.

Flaxseed oil tends to turn rancid very quickly, so it should be stored in your refrigerator. You can add the oil to cooked food, but do not use it during cooking because heat destroys its beneficial properties. Flaxseeds can be stored at room temperature for up to one year; ground seeds should be stored in your refrigerator in an airtight, opaque container.

Flaxseed oil also comes in capsules, but they are expensive compared to buying the bulk oil. Some health care practitioners and herbalists believe that flaxseed oil capsules, though convenient, are not as high quality as the pure oil because of the manufacturing process used to encapsulate them.

SIDE EFFECTS

No significant side effects or health hazards have been associated with consuming flaxseeds or flaxseed oil at the recommended therapeutic dosages. The absorption of drugs taken simultaneously with flaxseed may be delayed, so you should consult your health care practitioner or pharmacist about possible drug interactions if you are taking prescription medicine.

PERILLA OIL—AN UP-AND-COMING GOOD FAT

This rather obscure oil is derived from the seeds of the Asian beefsteak plant (*Perilla frutescens*), cultivated in Asian countries. Its leaves are used as a spice and in pickled food in Japan. No wonder, then, that most of the scientific research on perilla oil has been conducted in Japan. You can purchase perilla food products in the United States in many Korean grocery stores. Supplements made from the oil are available commercially in health food stores.

Perilla oil is packed with good fats and may even rival flaxseed oil in terms of its alpha-linolenic acid content, according to some analyses, making perilla oil one of nature's richest sources of omega-3s. The oil is also high in several *phenolic compounds,* natural chemicals that are therapeutically beneficial to health.

In Asia, herbalists prescribe perilla for relieving coughs, enhancing lung health, and fighting colds and flu. Various health claims have been attached to perilla oil, and these include its potential ability to fight allergies and asthma, ease pain and inflammation, stimulate immunity, and guard heart health. Some of these have been studied in research; others have not.

Whether perilla oil will be as beneficial as other healthful oils is not yet known, since very few clinical trials have been conducted with humans. Most of the research has been done in animals. Nonetheless, here's a look at what is currently known about this oil.

Treats Asthma

Affecting nearly 10 million Americans—most of them children—asthma is a serious, sometimes fatal disease. Its primary symptom is difficulty in breathing. During an asthma attack, antibodies react with allergens, producing histamine and other chemicals, which are responsible for most of the symptoms of asthma. Among the chemicals generated are pro-inflammatory leukotrienes.

In most cases, asthma is treated with inhaled medicine, oral doses of steroids and other drugs, and avoidance of allergens and pollutants. Recently though, perilla oil has been investigated as a potential treatment for asthma.

In one study, fourteen patients with asthma were randomly divided into two groups. For four weeks, one group supplemented with perilla oil; the other, with corn oil supplements. The findings: In the perilla oil–supplemented group, the generation of leukotrienes and other asthma-provoking substances was suppressed, whereas in the corn oil group, these chemicals increased. Lung function also improved in patients taking perilla oil. The researchers noted that perilla oil is useful for the treatment of asthma by suppressing substances that aggravate the disease and by strengthening breathing capacity.

Saves Hearts

Evidence is popping up that perilla oil may be good for your heart, according to researchers in Japan. They tested the effects of replacing soybean cooking oil with perilla oil (providing 3 grams a day of alpha-linolenic acid) in the diets of twenty elderly patients. The experiment worked like this: For six months, the subjects ate a diet enriched with soybean oil. After that, they consumed a diet enriched with perilla oil. Finally, they were switched back to the soybean oil–enriched diet so that researchers could compare the effects of the diets. The major finding of this study was that the 3-gram-a-day increase in alpha-linolenic acid caused the patients' bodies to churn out more EPA and DHA, both of which are heart-protective.

Perilla oil has also been shown to decrease abnormal blood clotting by 50 percent in studies of rodents. Lodged in an artery, a blood clot can narrow the passageway and choke off blood flow, leading to heart attack or stroke. Perilla oil appears to work in two ways: by reducing the production of platelet activating factor, a chemical released by cells that causes platelets (clotting elements in blood) to stick together; and by suppressing the production of thromboxane, another substance that makes platelets clump together and more apt to form clots.

Wards Off Cancer

Another potential plus for perilla oil: It may reduce the risk of colon cancer. In a Japanese experiment involving rats, researchers discovered that a small amount of perilla oil added to the diet (25 percent of total dietary fat) reduced the overall incidence of colon cancer in the animals. This led the researchers to note that perilla oil may help lower the risk of colon cancer.

In other animal studies, perilla oil has demonstrated an antitumor effect against tumors of the mammary gland and kidney.

Controls Weight

It may be just a blip on the research radar, but investigators in Japan discovered that perilla oil can shrink fat cells, prevent fat cells from enlarging (which results in obesity), and reduce the weight of fat pads in rats. The oil can also significantly reduce concentrations of triglycerides, or blood fats, in the animals. In their report, published in the *Journal of Nutrition,* the researchers wrote: "Therefore, daily consumption of perilla oil by humans seems advantageous."

It's certainly too early to tell whether perilla oil is a bona fide fat burner. However, these researchers are planning to study the antifat effect of perilla oil in humans—so stay tuned.

SUPPLEMENTING WITH PERILLA OIL

Perilla oil is available in supplements, and the typical daily dosage is around 6 grams, which provides 3 grams of alpha-linolenic acid. Dosage recommendations may vary from manufacturer to manufacturer, so read product labels for instructions. Check with your health care professional prior to supplementing with perilla oil.

SIDE EFFECTS

Most studies with perilla oil have been conducted with animals, so there is little information on its long-term safety in humans. Even so, perilla oil is widely consumed in a variety of Asian food products and has not been linked to any harmful side effects. Some health care practitioners recommend perilla oil over fish or flaxseed oil supplements because it is reportedly gentler on the stomach.

SIX

Omega-6 Healers

Although you should strive to pump up your omega-3 intake, you still need omega-6 fatty acids in your diet to help regulate and balance body processes. The key is to select better-quality omega-6 fats over inferior versions (generally found in margarine and processed foods). Higher-quality omega-6 oils include borage oil, black currant seed oil, and evening primrose oil, all of which can be used therapeutically to treat disease and strengthen health.

From this trio of oils, your body can directly obtain gamma-linolenic acid (GLA). In the body, GLA is also synthesized from the essential omega-6 fatty acid linoleic acid. GLA is ultimately metabolized into the prostaglandin E1 series, a group of beneficial chemicals that helps reduce inflammation, regulates blood clotting, decreases cholesterol levels, and lowers high blood pressure, among other functions.

Other omega-6 oils—namely sesame oil, wheat germ oil, and hempseed oil—are marketed as nutritional supplements. Some of these oils contain antioxidants and other substances beneficial to health. Here's a closer look at all of these omega-6 healers.

BORAGE: NATURE'S ALL-STAR OIL

*Some history: Borage is a plant that was originally cul-*tivated in Syria, and its name means "father of sweat" in Arabic, a reference to its use as a diaphoretic (an agent that increases perspiration). The ancient Romans were fond of borage, and Pliny the Elder recommended steeping it in wine to make a person more merry.

In folk medicine, borage has been used as a treatment for coughs and throat illnesses; as an anti-inflammatory agent for kidney, bladder, and joint problems; as a pain reliever; and as treatment for menopausal complaints.

Borage oil comes from the seeds of the borage plant and is a highly concentrated source of GLA, boasting 22 percent. A number of health conditions can benefit from treatment with GLA-rich borage oil.

Reduces Blood Pressure

A contributing factor to high blood pressure (hypertension) is stress in our lives. Happily, supplementing with borage oil may help you reduce stress-related high blood pressure, says a Canadian study. Researchers randomly assigned thirty men to one of three groups—borage oil supplements, fish oil supplements, and olive oil supplements—to see which supplements could reduce high blood pressure, provoked in response to a special type of test designed to induce stress. Borage oil alone kept blood pressure down, encouraged normal heart rate, and improved the subjects' performance on the test. Animal research also indicates that borage oil has a blood pressure–lowering effect.

Treats Respiratory Distress

Borage oil may save the lives of patients at risk for acute respiratory distress syndrome (ARDS). A common problem among patients in hospital intensive care units, ARDS kills approximately 50 percent of sufferers. The condition is associated with extensive lung inflammation and blood vessel injury in affected organs. ARDS comes on suddenly, and the lungs fill up with liquid. Patients drown in their own secretions.

Those at risk include trauma victims and patients with sepsis (internal infection), pneumonia, or shock, according to the American Lung Association. ARDS is also linked to extensive surgery, drowning, and inhalation of toxic gases. Conventional treatment consists of mechanical ventilation along with fluid removal and a special type of breathing technique.

A study of 150 at-risk patients at the Mayo Clinic found that borage oil reduced the mortality rate by 36 percent. Fluid samples taken from patients' lungs before and during treatment showed significantly lower white blood cell counts in those who were treated with borage oil, indicating reduced inflammation. The reason for the oil's healing effect: GLA, which reduces inflammation and improves oxygen flow in the body.

More studies are being conducted to confirm what doctors are beginning to suspect: that borage oil may improve the chances of recovery from ARDS.

Eases Rheumatoid Arthritis

More than 2 million people suffer from rheumatoid arthritis, a crippling autoimmune disease that strikes people of all ages, mostly women. Its symptoms include fever, joint stiffness and swelling, fatigue, muscle weakness, loss of appetite, and depression. Rheumatoid arthritis is "symmetrical" too, affecting the same joints on both sides of the body.

In rheumatoid arthritis, the body overproduces inflammation-producing chemicals, leading to the painful symptoms of the disease. Of all the plant oils, borage oil seems to work the best at soothing inflammation in this debilitating disease.

In a twenty-four-week clinical trial at the University of Pennsylvania, researchers treated thirty-seven rheumatoid arthritis patients with 1.4 grams a day of borage oil or cottonseed oil (the placebo). Treatment with borage oil produced some near-miraculous results: It reduced the number of tender joints by 36 percent and swollen joints by 28 percent. No such improvements were reported in the placebo takers. These findings led the researchers to state that borage oil was "a well-tolerated and effective treatment for active rheumatoid arthritis."

Borage oil may also benefit children with mild juvenile rheumatoid arthritis. In one study, children who took approximately 1 to 2 teaspoons of borage oil daily for a year experienced improved joint mobility, less morning stiffness, and fewer tender or swollen joints. They supplemented with borage oil in addition to their regular medicine, leading doctors to conclude that the oil may serve as an effective complementary treatment for juvenile rheumatoid arthritis.

USING BORAGE OIL

Herbalists suggest taking two to eight supplements of borage oil daily for its therapeutic benefits, but no more than 3 grams a day. You can also make a tea from the dried leaves of the borage plant. Add a cup of boiling water to about 2 teaspoons of dried leaves.

Borage oil should not be taken if you are taking anti-convulsants because it may interfere with the action of these drugs.

Borage oil is not appropriate for cooking because heat breaks down its chemical structure, and its fatty acids are converted to toxic by-products called lipid peroxides. Borage oil is best used as a medicinal oil.

It is important to add that borage is not approved by the German Commission E. One reason is that borage contains small amounts of plant chemicals called pyrrolizidine alkaloids (PA), which can contribute to liver damage and have been shown to be cancer-promoting in animal tests. That being the case, discuss the advisability of supplementation with your health care practitioner.

BLACK CURRANT SEED OIL: PRESCRIPTION FOR NATURAL HEALING

Black currant seed oil, derived from the seeds of the Ribes nigrum *plant grown in swamps and rain forests,* contains roughly 17 percent GLA and is one of nature's richest sources of this fatty acid. It is also a good source of the omega-3 fat alpha-linolenic acid, and thus provides a good balance of omega-6 and omega-3 fats.

What sets this oil apart is that it is the only com-

mercially available oil endowed with a fatty acid called
stearidonic acid, a by-product of alpha-linolenic acid. Investigators speculate that stearidonic acid is behind many
of the health benefits associated with black currant seed
oil.

Black currant seed oil has not been extensively researched; nonetheless, there is some evidence that it confers some important disease-fighting benefits.

Boosts Immunity

Supplementing with black currant seed oil may stimulate
your immune system, which tends to weaken with age. In
a study conducted at Tufts University, twenty-nine people
older than age sixty-five took 4.5 grams of black currant
seed oil or soybean oil (the placebo) every day for two
months. Researchers checked their immune function by
measuring their skin response to a toxin. Response to this
particular toxin generally declines with age.

By the end of the experimental period, those who supplemented with black currant seed oil showed a 28 percent
greater skin response than those on the placebo—which
meant that their immune systems had rallied to fight off
the toxin.

The researchers attributed the oil's immune-bolstering
effect to the ability of GLA to suppress the production of
prostaglandin E2, known to have an adverse effect on immune factors. Also, because older adults produce less
GLA, they may have benefited from supplementation with
a natural source of GLA.

Treats Rheumatoid Arthritis

Black currant seed oil is another fat that may be helpful in easing symptoms of rheumatoid arthritis. In one study, patients taking 525 milligrams of the oil every day experienced less morning stiffness.

Relieves Vaginal Dryness

Vaginal dryness occurs with age as vaginal tissues thin out, become less elastic, and stop secreting as much moisture. Herbalists suggest supplementing with black currant seed oil or other GLA-rich oils. The oil is believed to be important for the production of estrogen. Declining estrogen levels contribute to vaginal dryness.

Other Benefits

Research into the health benefits of black currant seed oil is under way, and preliminary findings, mostly with animals, show that it may also:

- Relieve diabetic nerve damage, a serious complication of diabetes

- Reduce high blood pressure

- Inhibit unhealthy blood clotting

- Suppress tumor growth

USING BLACK CURRANT SEED OIL

The recommended dosage of black currant seed oil ranges from two to eight capsules a day. Many health practitioners recommend taking no more than 4 grams a day.

Although there are no known side effects associated with taking black currant seed oil, check with your health care practitioner before deciding to supplement.

EVENING PRIMROSE OIL: NATURE'S ANSWER FOR WHAT AILS YOU

If your joints are creaky, your skin is dry and lifeless, or your menstrual symptoms are harder than ever to endure, don't despair. Reach for a gentle-on-your-body natural remedy called evening primrose oil, used down through the ages to treat a wide range of ailments.

Evening primrose oil comes from a plant that grows wild along roadsides. It is so named because its yellow flowers resemble real primroses, and these flowers open only in the evening.

The oil extracted from the seeds of this plant yields roughly 9 percent GLA, along with appreciable amounts of alpha-linolenic acid. Evening primrose oil is indicated for any diseases or conditions with which prostaglandins are associated, and these include premenstrual syndrome (PMS); heart disease; diabetic neuropathy, a type of nerve damage that is a complication of diabetes; and arthritis.

Evening primrose oil has long been used in Britain for treating women's health problems, particularly PMS. Here is a rundown of specific conditions for which evening primrose oil may be beneficial.

Eases Menstrual Symptoms

Among American Indian women, chewing the oil-rich seeds of the evening primrose plant is a centuries-old treatment for premenstrual and menstrual problems. And when 300 Australian women were asked to name their favorite treatments for PMS, the top three were dietary changes, vitamins, and evening primrose oil. What's more, evening primrose oil is an approved treatment for PMS in Great Britain.

And no wonder. This rather remarkable oil is an excellent alternative treatment for alleviating such symptoms as fluid retention, headaches and backaches, skin problems, food cravings, depression, tension, irritability, fatigue, weeping, tantrums, and lack of concentration.

Banishes Breast Pain

Supplementing with evening primrose oil may be the best way to ease breast pain (mastalgia) during menstruation. Painful breasts are a common menstrual and premenstrual problem that can range in severity from mild to severe pain. Mild breast pain, in fact, is considered normal and subsides when the woman's period is over.

Rest assured that breast pain is rarely a sign of cancer. Breast cancer–related pain tends to occur only in very-late-stage breast cancer, many years after treatment has started.

When breast pain is so severe that it interferes with daily living, many women often resort to prescription medications, either danazol (Danocrine) or bromocriptine. However, the side effects of these drugs can be worse than the breast pain itself. If you need relief, try evening primrose oil first. In studies, it has proven as effective as these drugs, but with no side effects. One study found that evening primrose oil was 97 percent effective against breast pain.

The reason it works so well is that many women with breast pain may be deficient in PGE1. A short supply of this prostaglandin intensifies the pain-inducing effect of another hormone, prolactin, on breast tissue. Evening primrose oil supplies extra GLA, which is ultimately converted to pain-relieving PGE1.

Acts as an Antioxidant

Among oilseeds, evening primrose has demonstrated some of the most powerful antioxidant activity. In one study, evening primrose oil snuffed out the hydroxyl radical, a form of hydrogen peroxide. Once generated, this devilish free radical attacks whatever is next to it, setting off a dangerous chain reaction that creates many more free radicals. In the same study, evening primrose reduced the formation of "superoxide" free radicals—a type of free radical that is particularly harmful to heart cells.

Cleans Out Arteries

Taking evening primrose oil may be one more weapon in your natural arsenal against high cholesterol. In a study of ten patients with high cholesterol, supplementation with 3.6 grams a day of evening primrose oil significantly reduced artery-clogging LDL cholesterol by 9 percent. Further, animal experiments show that evening primrose oil reduces plaque, which consists of fatty deposits that accumulate in arteries, narrow their passageways, and choke off blood flow.

Treats Diabetic Nerve Disease

Evening primrose oil has long been used as an alternative treatment for diabetes. One reason is that people with diabetes are often deficient in a special enzyme called delta-6-saturase, which is responsible for building many important components in the body. Without this enzyme, the body cannot convert the essential fatty acid linoleic acid into GLA. The impairment of such a critical enzyme creates a deficiency in essential fatty acid metabolism, which in turn leads to diabetic complications, primarily poor nerve conduction and sluggish blood flow in the extremities.

As noted earlier, evening primrose oil contains GLA. That's a plus because GLA does not require delta-6-saturase for breakdown by the body. Thus, some alternative health care practitioners believe that supplementation with evening primrose oil can supply needed amounts of GLA, circumvent an essential fatty acid deficiency, and thus help prevent diabetic complications.

Most of the research supporting this view has been conducted with animals, but the results are promising nonetheless. Nearly all of the studies have found that evening primrose oil corrects impaired nerve conduction and poor blood flow. In Germany, evening primrose oil is among the most widely recommended treatments for diabetic neuropathy.

Soothes Eczema

Because it lubricates your skin, evening primrose oil is an effective natural treatment for eczema, an inflammation of the skin that produces dryness, scaling, flaking, and itching. In clinical trials, evening primrose oil has been shown to reduce the severity of eczema and keep the skin smooth. As a result, many alternative health care practitioners recommend taking 500 milligrams of evening primrose oil each day to treat eczema. You should notice an improvement in your skin in about six to eight weeks.

The skin-smoothing benefits of evening primrose oil can be credited to GLA, which also has a hand in promoting healthy skin, hair, and nails. Scientists believe that the reason some people are prone to eczema is a defect in the enzyme delta-6-saturase, required for the conversion of linoleic acid to GLA. The body doesn't convert linoleic acid properly, resulting in a shortfall of GLA.

As explained before, supplementing with GLA-rich evening primrose oil circumvents this deficiency because GLA does not require the delta-6-saturase enzyme for breakdown by the body.

Combats Joint Problems

A growing number of medical experts and scientists now believe that taking GLA-rich oils such as evening primrose oil, borage oil, or black currant oil can effectively fight the inflammation—the major cause of swollen, painful joints—that is so characteristic of arthritis. As explained before GLA is a building block of the beneficial prostaglandin PGE1, which has an anti-inflammatory effect on the body. Thus, supplementing with GLA increases production of these prostaglandins and may help control the pain and inflammation associated with arthritis.

Fights Obesity

Evening primrose oil may be an antifat agent too. GLA, one of its beneficial constituents, has been researched for its involvement in weight loss in both animals and humans. In studies with rats, GLA reduced body fat content.

As for humans, some scientists believe that people with GLA deficiencies tend to produce more fat in their bodies. Supplementing with evening primrose oil has helped them lose weight.

Research has found that the supplement works best if you are more than 10 percent above your ideal weight. And, in some people, evening primrose oil promotes weight loss without reducing caloric intake. It is also believed to help rev up the metabolism so that you burn more calories.

Evening primrose oil helps reduce fluid retention, medically known as *edema*. When you retain water, you look and feel "fat," even though you aren't. Encouraging the body to get rid of extra water can make you look more trim. One way to do this is by supplementing with evening primrose oil, which can help your body regulate water more normally and prevent fluid retention.

Because of its potential antifat and anti-edema properties, evening primrose oil, along with grape-seed oil (another oil rich in omega-6 fats), is an ingredient in supplements designed to minimize cellulite. Cellulite is a cosmetic condition related to the deteriorating underlying structure of the skin. It is characterized by a lax, dimpled skin surface covering the thighs, buttocks, and hips. Grape-seed oil in particular may help improve circulation, strengthen connective tissue, and reduce fluid accumulation—all factors that improve the appearance of cellulite-ridden skin.

Kills Tumor Cells

In 1992, a group of researchers in India observed something quite exciting: that evening primrose oil killed tumor cells isolated in lab dishes. Why did the oil act like such a powerful terminator? The scientists chalked the effect up to the presence of linoleic acid and GLA in the oil, which may be able to slow down cancer.

In an animal study conducted by Welsh researchers, rats given evening primrose oil, fish oil, or a placebo oil were studied to determine the effect of these various oils on breast tumor growth. Breast tumors were significantly smaller in those animals fed evening primrose oil and fish oil.

Keep in mind that these experiments are not proof of an antitumor effect of evening primrose oil, only preliminary evidence. Without question, more studies are needed in this promising area of research.

Manages Migraines

More than 28 million Americans suffer from migraines—painful, often debilitating headaches that can last from hours to days or even weeks at a time. Migraine pain throbs, usually on one side of the head, or feels like a hammer pounding your head. Headaches are often accompanied by nausea and vomiting, as well as sensitivity to light and sound. About 20 percent of sufferers experience visual disturbances or auras prior to the actual migraine attack.

Headache specialists agree that migraine is a disorder of the central nervous system, but one that is not well understood. One theory holds that when something triggers a migraine, blood vessels in the head abnormally constrict and dilate, causing pain and inflammation. For this reason, herbalists recommend evening primrose oil to treat migraines because it is an anti-inflammatory agent that keeps blood vessels from constricting.

Some researchers believe that migraines can be alleviated by tinkering with essential fatty acid content in the diet. In a study conducted at the University of Berlin, 168 migraine sufferers supplemented with essential fatty acids for six months. The supplements contained 1,800 milligrams of GLA and alpha-linolenic acid. The patients were told to avoid high doses of arachidonic acid, found mostly in omega-6 fats. By the end of the study, 86 percent of the patients experienced a reduction in the severity, frequency, and duration of their migraine attacks, 90 percent had fewer incidents of nausea and vomiting, and 22 percent became migraine-free.

The researchers felt that the improvements came about in the following way: From both GLA and alpha-linolenic acid come inflammation-reducing prostaglandins and leukotrienes, and from arachidonic acid come prostaglandins and leukotrienes that step up inflammation. So by jacking up dietary levels of GLA and alpha-linolenic acid and cutting back on sources of arachidonic acid, the good prostaglandins and leukotrienes dominated in cells in order to produce an anti-inflammatory effect.

USING EVENING PRIMROSE OIL

No one knows yet what dosage of evening primrose oil is most beneficial. However, most alternative health care practitioners recommend a dosage of 1 to 4 grams a day, in divided doses, for general well-being. If you're treating breast pain, you may want to increase the dosage to 6 grams daily.

Evening primrose oil comes in softgel capsules. Typically, each capsule contains 500 milligrams of the oil and supplies 5 calories per capsule. Make sure the product supplies at least 45 milligrams (9 percent) of GLA per capsule.

Evening primrose oil appears to be safe, with very few side effects. Some potential side effects include stomach upset and headaches. As with any supplement, do not take evening primrose oil if you're pregnant or lactating.

SESAME OIL

The seeds of the sesame plant yield an abundant supply of omega-6 fats, disease-fighting antioxidants, and other therapeutic chemicals. A major component of the oil, for example, is an antioxidant called *sesaminol*. In experiments conducted in Japan, investigators observed that sesaminol worked better than vitamin E at guarding LDL cholesterol against free-radical–generated oxidation, which leads to artery damage. Based on this finding, they noted that "sesaminol is a potentially effective antioxidant that can protect LDL against oxidation." Sesame seeds also are rich in cholesterol-lowering compounds called *phytosterols* (plant steroids).

Sesame oil may also protect against stomach cancer. In Korea, where stomach cancer is the most prevalent form of malignancy, researchers at the Seoul National University College of Medicine have discovered that Koreans who frequently consume sesame oil have a decreased risk of stomach cancer. Other foods linked to a reduced risk included mung bean pancake, tofu, cabbage, and spinach.

There's more to the anticancer story: When exposed to sesame oil in test tubes, human colon cancer cells stopped growing and multiplying, according to a study conducted at Maharishi International University in Fairfield, Iowa. Other vegetable oils had a similar effect, although it was not as dramatic as that of sesame oil. The researchers pointed out that vegetable oils, including sesame oil, appear to have anticancer properties that warrant further investigation.

Applied topically, sesame oil is a therapeutic skin treatment widely used in Ayurveda (pronounced *eye-yuhr-VAY-dah*), a system of medicine used for more than 5,000 years in India. Ayurveda treats diseases holistically, with nutrition, exercise, meditation, and other lifestyle-management approaches. In another study at Maharishi International University, researchers observed that sesame oil, as well as safflower oil, inhibited the growth of malignant melanoma cells in lab dishes. Malignant melanoma is the deadliest form of skin cancer.

Sesame oil is used mostly in cooking and is a popular oil for preparing Asian dishes. A note of caution: Sesame seeds and sesame oil contain allergens, which can provoke an allergic reaction in susceptible people.

WHEAT GERM AND WHEAT GERM OIL

At the heart of a kernel of wheat grain is the germ, or the sprouting portion of the kernel. It's an excellent source of vitamin E, protein, B-complex vitamins, and various minerals, including calcium, magnesium, phosphorus, copper, and manganese. Wheat germ is usually removed from the grain during milling because its fat content can turn the flour rancid. Wheat germ oil is extracted from wheat germ and sold as a nutritional supplement. Fifty-eight percent of the essential fatty acids in the oil are omega-6 fats. Wheat germ oil is also high in vitamin E, an important antioxidant.

From wheat germ oil comes the supplement octacosanol, an alcohol derivative of the oil. Athletes have long used octacosanol in the belief that it will improve energy, strength, and reaction time, although no research has turned up any proof that it directly improves endurance or physical performance. Some studies suggest that octacosanol may help regulate cholesterol and prevent platelet stickiness (which can lead to abnormal blood clotting).

There are no known adverse reactions or side effects to using wheat germ, wheat germ oil, or octacosanol. In fact, wheat germ is an excellent, nutrient-packed food to include in the diet, although it is rather high in calories (360 calories in a 3 ½-ounce serving).

Wheat germ oil is available in capsules and in liquid form. Follow the manufacturer's suggest dosage if you decide to supplement with wheat germ oil.

HEMPSEED OIL

You may have heard or read about a nutritional oil called hempseed oil. It is extracted from the seeds of the hemp plant, also the source of the narcotic marijuana. But you won't get high from hempseed oil. Recently, newer hemp cultivars have been developed that yield a seed that is practically devoid of THC (tetrahydrocannabinol), the narcotic in hemp.

Still, it is illegal to grow the hemp plant in the United States, so hempseed oil is manufactured mostly in Canada, the United Kingdom, and parts of Asia and imported for

use in cosmetics and toiletries. Hempseed oil is also available as a dietary supplement from various companies that
market nutritional oils.

Hempseed oil is loaded with essential fats: omega-6 fats
(58 percent), omega-3 fats (20 percent), monounsaturated
fats (11 percent), and GLA (1 to 3 percent).

There have been very few studies conducted on the
health benefits of hempseed oil, however, so it is not yet
known whether it can be used effectively to treat diseases
that benefit from essential fatty acid supplements.

A red flag: If you consume hempseed oil, you may test
positive in a urine drug test for metabolites called cannabinoids, which are also evident in urine after marijuana
use.

PART III.

More Good-for-You Fats

SEVEN

Olive Oil:
The Master Monounsaturated Fat

You're lunching on a Greek salad, built on a bed of green, leafy lettuce piled high with tomatoes, olives, and crumbled feta cheese. The salad is drizzled with a dressing made from extra-virgin olive oil with some vinegar and spices thrown in for added zing. With each forkful, you're plying your body with oleic acid, squalene, oleuropein, hydroxytyrosol, tyrosol, and other substances with hard-to-pronounce names.

Sound unappetizing? Don't let these names scare you. They designate an array of healthy food components, all with some amazing disease-fighting properties. You happen to be lunching on a combination of foods that has been eaten for hundreds of years in the Mediterranean, where rates of heart disease and cancer are among the lowest on the planet.

The so-called Mediterranean diet refers to the cuisine eaten primarily in Greece and southern Italy. It is characterized by low consumption of red meat; lots of fruits, vegetables, and grains; moderate amounts of red wine;

and loads of olive oil. In fact, the fats derived from olive oil make up more than a third of the total daily calories for people from these countries. In Greece alone, the diet provides up to 42 percent of its calories as fat, primarily from olives and olive oil. Despite their high-fat eating habits, Greeks living in Greece enjoy the longest life expectancies of any group of people in the world.

But so healthy is the Mediterranean diet that from decades of research, it appears that if you eat like this, you're least likely to die of anything (with the exception of very old age). And olive oil is a prime reason.

What's so special about olive oil?

Rich in monounsaturated fats, olive oil has been used for centuries to maintain the suppleness of skin, give sheen to hair, aid in digestion, relieve muscle pain, and lower blood pressure. Ancient Egyptians used olive oil for preserving mummies, and the Bible mentions the oil frequently as a medicine for healing wounds and anointing the sick.

Among unsaturated fats, olive oil stands alone as being resistant to oxidation, a possible factor in heart disease. Because of this attribute, olive oil has been described as the safest fat to eat because it doesn't readily oxidize and give off health-damaging free radicals. More recently, olive oil has been shown to conserve heart-protective HDL cholesterol. Further, olive oil also seems to guard Mediterranean people from certain forms of cancer, specifically cancers of the colon, breast, endometrium, and prostate. Another plus for olive oil: Antioxidant vitamin E does a better job of fighting off free radicals if olive oil is present in your diet.

The secret to olive oil's power lies in its host of healthy constituents mentioned earlier. Let's return to those funny-sounding names for a moment and delve into what they do so you can understand the powerful effect they can have on your health.

OLEIC ACID: A DISEASE-STOPPING FATTY ACID

The chief monounsaturated fatty acid in olives and olive oil is an omega-9 fatty acid called *oleic acid*, which constitutes 80 percent of the oil. Oleic acid is also distributed in canola (see Table 8 in this chapter), almond, avocado, canola, peanut, safflower, and sunflower oils. It is what gives all of these oils, including olive oil, their ability to withstand higher cooking temperatures. So healthy is oleic acid that other vegetable oils have been specially modified to pump up their content of this fatty acid. Examples include high-oleic sunflower oil and high-oleic soybean oil. There is also an appreciable amount of oleic acid in meat, but the huge amounts of saturated fat in meat cancel out any good health deeds its oleic acid might do.

The high percentage of oleic acid in olive oil protects your cardiovascular health and may decrease your risk of heart attack and stroke, according to a growing body of research. Specifically, oleic acid in olive oil:

- Influences blood levels of harmful LDL cholesterol (the lower your intake of oleic acid, the higher your LDL cholesterol levels)

- Increases levels of protective HDL cholesterol

- Blocks the abnormal buildup of fat and plaque in arteries, which can lead to atherosclerosis, the narrowing and thickening of artery walls

* Lowers triglycerides, a blood fat that in excessive amounts can contribute to heart disease

Olive oil clearly does your heart good. So if you're interested in preventing and treating heart disease, include olive oil as one of the main good fats in your diet.

SQUALENE: SECRET CANCER-FIGHTING INGREDIENT

Olive oil is well endowed with a vitaminlike chemical called *squalene*. Squalene is also present in shark liver oil and human sebum, an oily secretion that lubricates your skin.

Some rather fascinating statistics: The average intake of squalene in the United States is 30 milligrams a day, whereas in Mediterranean countries, the typical intake is 200 to 400 milligrams a day. Because of this dietary disparity, many scientists feel that the low incidence of cancer in Mediterranean countries is somehow linked to the higher intake of squalene obtained through olive oil.

Indeed, experiments with squalene show that it inhibits colon, lung, and skin tumors in rodents. Squalene is believed to work by suppressing the action of a key enzyme required for the growth of cancer cells. To date, no human studies have been conducted on the anticancer effect of squalene, although some scientists are convinced that this chemical may turn out to be the true cancer fighter in olive oil.

But with regard to colon cancer, a team of researchers at the Institute of Health Sciences in Britain compared colon cancer rates, diets, and olive oil consumption in twenty-eight countries, including Europe, Britain, the

United States, Brazil, Colombia, Canada, and China. They discovered that countries with a diet high in meat and low in vegetables had the highest rates of colon cancer. But olive oil was associated with a lower risk, leading the researchers to conclude that olive oil may have a protective effect on the development of colon cancer. The study didn't single out squalene as the reason, but as previously noted, other scientists have emphasized that it could be responsible for the cancer-fighting effect of olive oil.

Among squalene's other functions in the body are to act as an intermediate, or a go-between, in the synthesis of cholesterol. In essence, it helps regulate how much cholesterol is made and may even inhibit the abnormal production of this fatty substance. In a study of elderly patients, the combination of squalene (860 milligrams) with a cholesterol-lowering drug called pravastatin (10 milligrams) did a better job of lowering harmful LDL cholesterol and increasing beneficial HDL cholesterol than treatment with the drug by itself.

OLEUROPEIN: SPECIAL ANTIOXIDANT POWERS

Technically, oleuropein *is a polyphenol, a term that de-*scribes its chemical structure. Distributed widely in plant foods, polyphenols are disease-fighting substances that boast a lengthy resume of health-promoting accomplishments, particularly in cardiovascular health and cancer protection. They are also responsible for the characteristic stability of olive oil, preventing it from turning rancid.

Oleuropein is the most abundant polyphenol in olives and olive oil. It gives olives their bitter taste, but more important, it acts as a mighty antioxidant to snuff out harmful free radicals. Experiments show that oleuropein can squelch the superoxide radical, a nasty molecule that inflicts tissue injury by damaging structural lipids in cell membranes. What's more, oleuropein can shut down a dangerous free-radical–generating process in the body.

There is mounting interest in oleuropein as a cholesterol fighter. In lab dishes, it has demonstrated potent antioxidant activity against the oxidation of LDL cholesterol—a process initiated by free radicals. When LDL is oxidized by free radicals, white blood cells in artery linings start attracting excessive amounts of LDL. The oxidized LDL forms lesions on the inner arterial walls, and cholesterol is deposited in these lesions—a process that leads to atherosclerosis.

There's more: Oleuropein appears to keep body-invading bacteria at bay, say investigators at the University of Messina in Italy. They found that oleuropein curbed the growth of various bacterial strains, specifically those that attack the intestines and urinary tract.

HYDROXYTYROSOL: A FREE-RADICAL ATTACKER

Another powerful antioxidant in olives and olive oil is a polyphenol called *hydroxytyrosol,* a biological "chip off the old block," formed when it splits from oleuropein during an enzyme-controlled reaction. In the body, hydroxytyrosol combines forces with oleuropein, creating a dynamic antioxidant duo that is more powerful against free radicals than even vitamin C, another potent antioxidant.

Separately, hydroxytyrosol is an effective antioxidant in its own right. An interesting study conducted with rats at the University of Milan found that hydroxytyrosol prevented oxidative stress caused by exposure to passive smoking. Oxidative stress is a harmful condition that occurs when free radicals outnumber antioxidants in the body. Quite possibly, eating olive oil may fortify your bodily defenses against the adverse health effects linked to secondhand smoke.

Like oleuropein, hydroxytyrosol prevents the dangerous oxidation of LDL cholesterol and suppresses abnormal blood clotting—two benefits that make this healthful chemical a worthy dietary defense against heart disease.

Also, a recent Italian study discovered that hydroxytyrosol stopped cultured leukemia cells from multiplying and caused them to "commit suicide." This is very preliminary research, but promising nonetheless.

TYROSOL: HEART HELPER

The third major polyphenol in olives and olive oil is tyrosol. Like its companion polyphenols, tyrosol is an antioxidant that prevents the oxidation of LDL cholesterol and keeps free radicals from attacking cell membranes.

Tyrosol may have anticancer properties as well. In one study, researchers in Italy discovered that tyrosol protected human colon cells in lab dishes from turning cancerous in response to oxidation.

Many scientists believe that tyrosol and the other polyphenols in olive oil have blood pressure–lowering properties. In one study, patients with high blood pressure who followed an olive oil–enriched diet were able to discontinue taking their blood pressure pills.

Why does tyrosol have such a profound benefit? Researchers chalk it up to the antioxidant effect of polyphenols against free radicals. The production of free radicals blocks the production of nitric oxide, a blood vessel relaxant that helps keep blood pressure down. Thus, eating more polyphenols—including those from olive oil—may help keep your blood pressure in check.

MAXIMIZE THE HEALTH BENEFITS OF OLIVE OIL

Here's something else you should know: You can get even more health-protecting power from olive oil by adding it to tomato-based recipes. That's because combining olive oil with tomato products soups up the protective powers of lycopene, an antioxidant that may help prevent heart disease and cancer. In a study comparing the addition of olive oil versus sunflower oil to tomato products, only the mixture of olive oil with tomato increased antioxidant activity.

PURCHASING OLIVE OIL

There is a dizzying array of various types of olive oil on supermarket shelves: extra-virgin olive oil, fine virgin olive oil, virgin olive oil, light olive oil, and so on. Not only that, olive oils are manufactured in more than twenty-two different countries, with widely different soil conditions, and are extracted from a large variety of olives, each with its own characteristics. All of these factors account for huge variations in the fatty acid and nutrient content of olive oil.

That being the case: Which olive oil is best, and does it even matter?

Some olive oils are healthier and more potent than others, so it does matter which type you buy. Basically, olive oils differ in their concentration of fatty acids and antioxidants—a difference largely due to the oil extraction process. The less heat and fewer chemicals used to extract the oil, the more nutritious the olive oil is.

Olive oil contains 115 calories per tablespoon—approximately the same number found in other cooking or salad oils. You may be able to save calories, however, because olive oil has a greater flavor and aroma than other oils, and that means you can use less when cooking. Olive oil is also cholesterol-free.

Table 7 provides a comparison of the various types of olive oil available.

Clearly, your best bet is extra-virgin olive oil. But even then, there are differences in levels of two important components: oleic acid and squalene.

Some cancer researchers feel that the ratio of oleic acid to linoleic acid, an omega-6 fatty acid, is the best indicator of an olive oil's cancer-fighting power. A higher proportion of oleic acid to linoleic acid is considered desirable. As noted, other researchers feel that the squalene in olive oil is responsible for its anticancer benefit.

In 1999, *Prevention Magazine,* a leading health publication, tested various extra-virgin olive oils for their ratio of oleic acid to linoleic acid and for their squalene content. In an article published in the September 1999 issue, writer Mike McGrath reported that olive oils from Spain, Italy, and Greece scored the highest for oleic acid ratios and squalene content. As for squalene, one oil stood out for having the highest amount of this protective nutrient: St. Helene Extra Virgin, an olive oil made in California.

Best advice: Buy extra-virgin olive oil, preferably from

Table 7

PROPERTIES AND USES OF OLIVE OIL

Type	Processing Method	Color/Taste	Uses	Healthful Properties
Extra-virgin	Obtained from the first pressing of the ripe fruit by mechanical and physical methods. No heat or chemicals are used. The only vegetable oil that is not chemically processed.	Pale yellow to bright green; fruity taste; wide range of flavors and aromas.	Salad dressings; dipping bread.	Contains all the fatty acids and antioxidants found in the olives from which it is made. High levels of squalene. The only edible oil that contains polyphenols. Appears to be more protective against LDL oxidation than other olive oils.
Virgin	A second-press oil; however, some are processed using chemicals.	Colorless; good flavor.	Salad dressings; dipping bread; cooking. (Not widely available in the United States.)	Contains a negligible amount of polyphenols and squalene.
Fine	A blend of extra-virgin and virgin olive oils.	Varies in level of fruitiness.	Salad dressings; dipping bread; cooking.	Combines some of the nutrient characteristics of extra-virgin and virgin olive oils.

Table 7 continued

PROPERTIES AND USES OF OLIVE OIL

Type	Processing Method	Color/Taste	Uses	Healthful Properties
Pure olive oil	Produced by chemically extracting oil from the remaining pulp left over after cold-pressing.	Yellow to green; tasteless.	A general-purpose olive oil.	Contains little or no healthful substances.
Light	This is pure olive oil blended with a tiny amount of extra-virgin olive oil.	Lightest in color of all olive oils; generally tasteless. ("Light" or "lite" refers to color, not caloric content. All olive oils contain roughly the same amount of calories.)	Recommended for cooking.	Contains the same amount of beneficial monounsaturates as other olive oils, but contains few other healthful substances.

Mediterranean countries, or check out the California-made oil mentioned earlier to reap the health-protective benefits of this exceptionally good fat.

See Table 8 for a discussion of another healthy monounsaturated fat: canola oil.

Table 8

THE OTHER MIGHTY MONOUNSATURATE

Another good fat with plenty of virtues is canola oil. Among cooking oils, it contains the lowest level (6 percent) of artery-clogging saturated fat and boasts 61 percent of heart-healthy oleic acid, making it second only to olive oil in oleic acid content. There are also considerable amounts of linoleic acid (22 percent), an omega-6 fatty acid, and alpha-linolenic acid (11 percent), an omega-3 fatty acid, in canola oil.

Canola oil is pressed from the seeds of the rapeseed plant, a relative of the mustard plant that has been cultivated in China and India for more than 4,000 years. Originally, oil from the rapeseed plant was available as a food oil solely in Europe and Canada, but not in the United States because it was accused of causing heart abnormalities in rats and consigned to industrial uses only. A new cultivar of the plant was bred to be very low in a natural but potentially toxic fatty acid called erudic acid, and in 1985, its oil was approved by the FDA for cooking. The FDA considers the low erudic acid content (0.6) of canola oil safe for human consumption.

At first, the oil was required to be labeled "low-erudic-acid rapeseed oil," but in 1988, the FDA permitted the product to be called canola oil, the name used in Canada, where most of the oil is produced. In the United States, some canola oil is made in Indiana, Kentucky, and Tennessee.

Like olive oil and many other good fats, canola oil has been found in research to lower total cholesterol and LDL cholesterol and normalize the clotting activity of platelets, thereby reducing the risk of heart disease. In animal studies, it has been shown to protect against dangerous arrhythmias (irregular heartbeats).

Canola oil contains 120 calories per tablespoon, is available as cooking oil, and is found in margarines.

EIGHT

The New Heart-Saving Fats

Attention spread lovers: Want to have your margarine and butter—and eat it too? Then check out the margarine spreads Benecol and Take Control, which are designed specifically to reduce cholesterol levels in the blood.

In 1999, the U.S. Food and Drug Administration (FDA) approved both products with the designation *functional foods*. Technically, the term *functional food* refers to a food product that is beneficial to health. In its position paper on functional foods, the American Dietetic Association formally defines such foods as "any modified food or food ingredient that may provide a health benefit beyond the traditional nutrients it contains." Benecol and Take Control fit this definition because they are formulated with ingredients designed to improve cardiovascular health.

Both margarines are predominantly monounsaturated fats (mainly canola oil) fortified with plant sterols, including *sterol esters* and *stanol esters*. Similar in structure to cholesterol found in animals, plant sterols are present in small quantities in many fruits, vegetables, legumes, nuts, seeds, grains, and other plant sources. Benecol contains plant stanol esters from a compound found in pinewood pulp, and Take Control uses plant sterol esters extracted from soybean oil. If your cholesterol is moderately high, Benecol and Take Control may help you control it, reducing your risk of artery damage.

HOW CHOLESTEROL-LOWERING MARGARINES WORK

*Under normal conditions, LDL cholesterol delivers choles-*terol to cells to make cell membranes, sex hormones, and other substances. But in excessive amounts, LDL cholesterol—the so-called bad cholesterol—can lead to artery damage. By contrast, HDL cholesterol—known as the good cholesterol—picks up cholesterol from cells and shuttles it to the liver, where the cholesterol is turned into bile acids (*biliary cholesterol*) and secreted in the intestines.

Essentially, plant sterols make it harder for your intestines to absorb cholesterol from the small intestine. Plus, they increase the excretion of both biliary cholesterol and dietary cholesterol.

Specifically, plant sterols work in the following manner: When your body soaks up cholesterol from the small intestine, the cholesterol is first wrapped in a *micelle,* a tiny droplet made of lipids and emulsifiers from bile. Because plant stanol/sterol esters are very similar in shape to cholesterol, micelles mistake them for cholesterol. If a plant stanol/sterol ester gets into the micelle first, there's no room for cholesterol. In essence, plant sterols and cholesterol compete for entry into the micelles. Unable to enter the micelle, cholesterol is blocked from absorption into the bloodstream. The net effect of displacing cholesterol is reduced levels of LDL cholesterol in the blood and the preservation of levels of HDL cholesterol. Cholesterol-lowering margarines do not raise HDL cholesterol, block saturated fat, or lower triglycerides, however.

A LOOK AT THE SCIENTIFIC PROOF

Have these products been scientifically proven to reduce cholesterol? Yes. Here's the scoop:

- A yearlong study conducted at the University of Helsinki in Finland compared patients using Benecol with patients using regular margarine (the control group). Benecol (roughly 2 tablespoons eaten daily for one year) reduced overall cholesterol levels by 10 percent and LDL cholesterol by 14 percent in people whose cholesterol was mildly elevated (between 200 mg/dl and 240 mg/dl). What this means: Let's say your total cholesterol is 230; eating Benecol could lower it by as much as 23 points.

  As for Take Control, research shows that it cuts LDL cholesterol by 10 percent, when patients used one or two pats a day, and by 17 percent when used as part of a heart-healthy diet.

- For more dramatic results, try combining cholesterol-lowering spreads with cholesterol-lowering drugs called *statins* (but check with your physician first). Statins lower LDL cholesterol by curtailing your body's production of cholesterol.

In twenty-two women diagnosed with heart disease, Benecol alone dropped total cholesterol by 13 percent and LDL cholesterol by 20 percent. Combined with a statin drug, Benecol cut cholesterol levels even further: total cholesterol by an extra 11 percent and LDL cholesterol by an extra 16 percent in just twelve weeks.

In a third of the women tested, Benecol alone normalized cholesterol. In others, the combination of Benecol and the statin drug was found to be more effective than the statin alone. What's more, the combo allowed some patients to take a lower dosage of medication, and in some cases, eliminated the need for the drug altogether. This is certainly good news, since statins often have side effects, including liver problems, stomach upset, and muscle pain.

These findings are monumentally significant for women. Here's why: If you're like most women, you probably think heart disease is a "guy thing"—you know, like football, hunting, or John Wayne movies. But that perception is not only false, it's dangerous. Among women, heart disease claims more lives than all forms of cancer combined, even breast cancer. Statistics show that heart disease strikes 36 percent of women, while breast cancer affects 4 percent. One in two women will die from a first heart attack, compared to one in four men. And among those who do survive, 20 percent will have a second heart attack within four years, compared to 16 percent of men. The study cited earlier simply means that now women have one more weapon—plant stanol/sterol esters—to get their cholesterol levels under control and defend themselves against heart disease.

So that men don't feel left out: Benecol (5.1 grams a day) reduced total cholesterol by 12 percent and LDL cholesterol by 17 percent in men (and women) undergoing statin therapy but who still had elevated LDL cholesterol, according to an eight-week study conducted at the Cooper Institute in Dallas, Texas.

- Plant sterols complement the cholesterol-lowering effects of a low-fat diet, which is recommended as a way to reduce cholesterol. Studies show that people who strictly adhere to low-fat eating, can slash cholesterol by 15 to 37 percent. Often, though, it's tough to stick to a low-fat diet because fat—especially the saturated variety—is so hard to give up.

  If that sounds all too familiar, swap your favorite fats such as margarine and butter for a product such as Benecol or Take Control. In a study conducted at the University of Kuopio in Finland, people who ate wood- or vegetable-derived plant sterols while following a low-fat diet brought their total cholesterol and LDL cholesterol down even lower than by following a low-fat diet alone.

  What constituted a low-fat diet in this study? The experimental diet provided 28 to 30 percent of total calories from fat (8 to 10 percent as saturated fat, 12 percent as monounsaturated fat, and 8 percent as polyunsaturated fat), 20 percent of calories from protein, and 50 to 52 percent from carbohydrates.

- Benecol and Take Control work equally well. A study of ninety-five patients conducted in the Netherlands compared the effects of margarines fortified with either plant stanol esters or plant sterol esters. Both types of margarines brought total cholesterol and LDL cholesterol down by as much as 8 to 13 percent.

- Plant sterols may turn out to be effective dietary tools

for heading heart disease off at the pass, even reversing its course. Based on the expected LDL cholesterol reduction of 10 to 14 percent, scientists estimate that plant sterols may be able to cut the risk of heart disease by a whopping 25 percent. Already, in experiments with mice, plant sterols have inhibited the formation of lesions inside artery walls, reversing the development of atherosclerosis. Of course, we need more research, particularly with humans, to see how this all shakes out, but plant sterols certainly show enormous potential in preventing heart disease.

USING CHOLESTEROL-LOWERING MARGARINES

Benecol and Take Control most definitely count as healthy fats. The fact that they are made from monounsaturated fats is a plus because mono fats are practically immune to oxidation, a factor in atherosclerosis.

It should be noted that Benecol contains minute amounts of trans-fatty acids—less than 0.5 grams per 8-gram serving. (Foods totaling less than 0.5 grams can claim to be transfree.) Take Control contains 0 grams of trans-fatty acids per serving.

Here are some additional tips for using these products to your best advantage:

+ With Benecol, the manufacturer (McNeil Consumer Healthcare) recommends three daily servings (½ teaspoons each) to move your cholesterol into a healthier range. Two servings a day (2 tablespoons) of Take Control are recommended by its manufacturer (Lipton).

- You can use these products at a single meal or divide your servings over three meals. A recent study demonstrated that a daily serving of 2.5 grams of plant stanol esters eaten once at lunch lowered LDL cholesterol just as effectively as spreading the serving over three meals (0.42 grams at breakfast, 0.84 grams at lunch, and 1.25 grams at dinner). These findings suggest that plant sterols stay in the intestinal tract for several hours after meals.

- These spreads should always be used in place of—not in addition to—butter or margarine. You can spread them on toast, vegetables, crackers, potatoes, bagels, or other favorite foods.

- Try cooking, baking, or frying with Benecol Regular Spread. Take Control is not recommended for cooking.

- Benecol and Take Control come in tubs, like other margarines in use today, making it easy to measure out portions.

- Figure these margarines into your daily calorie count if you're watching your weight. Benecol Regular contains 45 calories per serving; Benecol Light, 30 calories per serving. Take Control contains 50 calories per serving; Take Control Light, 40 calories per serving.

- Use these products as part of an overall cholesterol-reduction program that includes eating less saturated fat and trans-fatty acids, exercising, quitting smoking, losing weight, and taking cholesterol-lowering drugs, if prescribed. Benecol is also available in snack bars and salad dressings.

- Eating more than the recommended amount will not

lower cholesterol more than the 10 to 14 percent observed in studies.

- While these products are effective for fighting elevated cholesterol, they can also be used by anyone who wants to guard against too-high cholesterol.

- Cholesterol-lowering spreads have been intensely evaluated for safety and have passed with flying colors, earning the Generally Recognized As Safe (GRAS) designation from the FDA.

Table 9

What Are Fake Fats?

Plant stanol/sterol esters are not the same substances as *fat replacers*. Fat replacers are additives concocted from carbohydrates, protein, and other fats to trick your mouth into believing you're getting a high-fat treat, but without the calories. They resemble fats in all ways except two: They don't plug arteries, and they're low in calories.

Fat replacers and fat substitutes are categorized as follows:

- **Carbohydrate-based fats.** Formulated from starches and fibers, carbohydrate-based fats are used in frozen desserts, puddings, cake frostings, margarines, and salad dressings to replace the real fat. Examples include polydextrose, a partially absorbable starch that supplies about 1 calorie per gram (versus 9 calories per gram from fat), and maltodextrin, a starch made from corn. Cellulose and gum are two types of fibers used to manufacture fat replacers. When ground into tiny particles, cellulose forms a consistency that feels like fat when eaten. Cellulose replaces some or all of the fat in certain dairy-type products, sauces, frozen desserts, and salad dressings. Gums such as xanthan gum, guar gum, pectin, and carrageenan are used to thicken foods and give them a creamy texture. Added to salad dressings, desserts, and processed meats, gums cut the fat content considerably. Side effects of carbohydrate-based fat replacers include gas, bloating, and cramping.

- **Protein-based fat replacers.** These are formulated from milk or eggs, created by heating and blending milk or egg white proteins into mistlike particles—technically known as *microparticulated protein*. Like real fat, these processed proteins feel creamy on the tongue. You'll want to avoid this type of fat replacer if you are allergic to milk or eggs.

- **Fat-based fat replacers.** When serving a fattening dessert, have you ever jokingly told your guests that "all the calories have been taken out"? It can be done! Food technologists can chemically change the properties of fats to remove or drastically cut fat calories. The result is fat-based fat replacers and fat substitutes. Some pass through the body unabsorbed, making them calorie-free. Others can even be used in cooking and frying, unlike carbohydrate- and protein-based fat replacers.

  One of these is Olestra from Procter & Gamble. Technically, Olestra is a *sucrose polyester,* meaning a combination of sugar and fatty acids. Your body can't digest Olestra, so it's classified as a noncaloric product.

  According to the manufacturer, Olestra can be substituted for fats and oils in foods without loss of flavor. It has the same cooking properties as fats and oils and can be used in shortenings, oils, margarines, ice creams, desserts, and snacks. Also, Olestra may block the absorption of vitamins A, D, E, and K. Side effects include cramping and loose stools.

  Other fat-based fat replacers are emulsifiers, which reduce fat and calories by replacing the shortening in cake mixes, cookies, icings, and other products, and caprenin, a cocoa butter–like ingredient used in candy.

- **Combinations.** Some fat replacers are formulated from a combination of carbohydrates, proteins, and fats. Combination-type fat replacers are found ice cream, salad oils, mayonnaise, spreads, sauces, and bakery products.

  The key to enjoying any new fat-free product is to include it in your diet using a tried-and-true nutrition maxim—with moderation. Remember too that even though a food may be fat-free, it's not necessarily calorie-free. If you eat a lot of fat-free products, you could be overconsuming calories and packing on pounds as a result.

PART IV

The Fat-Burning Fats

NINE

Conjugated Linoleic Acid: Health Insurance in a Pill

Talk about confusing: Some fats have been linked to the most life-threatening diseases on the face of the earth— heart disease, cancer, diabetes, and obesity. Even so, there is yet another fat that has the power to prevent and treat the very same diseases!

How can this be?

Meet conjugated linoleic acid (CLA), another body-friendly fat that provides excellent health insurance against a variety of ills. Discovered in 1978 at the University of Wisconsin, CLA is a naturally occurring fatty acid present in dairy products (most notably, milk fat), as well as in meat, sunflower oil, and safflower oil. It is formed when the bacteria in a cow's gut breaks down the essential fatty acid, linoleic acid, in the food the animal eats.

In 1996, CLA became available as a diet product derived from sunflower oil. Ads for CLA note that the nutrient may be missing from many diets (presumably since some people tend to eat less meat and high-fat dairy products). Since its discovery, there has been an explosion of research on CLA—all pointing to some rather amazing results, particularly in the area of weight loss and weight management.

Here's a rundown on the health-protecting properties of this rather remarkable supplement. CLA:

Melts Pounds

At any given time, 33 to 40 percent of women and 20 to 24 percent of men are trying to knock off pounds, says the American Society of Bariatric Physicians (physicians who specialize in weight loss). Wouldn't it be great if we could pop a pill to melt fat, but experience no untoward side effects? CLA may very well be that pill.

Much research with animals documents that CLA is a potent fat-fighter. In tests with mice, CLA pared down body fat (even at night), curbed appetite, boosted metabolism—and spot-reduced the animals' abdominal area!

Although the mechanism of CLA's fat-fighting action is unclear, researchers have found that it encourages the breakdown of fat, stifles a fat storage enzyme called *lipoprotein lipase,* and kills off fat cells. All three factors could be responsible for CLA's fat-burning benefits—at least in animals.

Some researchers believe that CLA may interact with *cytokines,* proteins that are involved in energy production and fat metabolism. They theorize that CLA somehow causes dietary protein, carbohydrates, and fats to be used by cells for energy and muscle tissue growth, rather than be stored as fat.

Another observation: CLA investigators say that the supplement does not shrink fat cells (like weight-loss diets do), but rather, it keeps them from enlarging. Enlarged fat cells are the main reason we get pudgy.

But does CLA work as well in humans? A string of new evidence from human trials shows that while CLA will not decrease your body weight, it does something better: It reduces body fat and builds body-firming muscle. Muscle is metabolically active, meaning that it burns fat even while you're resting. Also, the more muscle you have, the faster your metabolism. A fast metabolism translates into better weight loss and better weight control.

In one study, conducted at the University of Wisconsin in Madison, volunteers took 3 grams of CLA for six months. The findings showed that CLA kept people from gaining weight, and also increased their muscle tissue. That's good news for people entering middle age. Here's why: We tend to get fatter and lose muscle with age; thus, supplementing with CLA just might prevent middle-age spread.

In a study at Kent State University twenty-four men, ages nineteen to twenty-eight, supplemented with either 7.2 grams a day of CLA, or a vegetable oil placebo, while participating in a six-week bodybuilding program. The CLA-supplementers experienced gains in the following areas: greater arm girth, overall body mass, and improved leg strength. The researchers commented that "apparently CLA acts as a mild anabolic agent."

In another human study, twenty nonobese people (ten men and ten women) were given just over a gram of CLA or a placebo with breakfast, lunch, and dinner. They were instructed not to change their diet or exercise habits.

At the end of three months, the researchers measured both the weight and body fat percentage of the study participants. Even though there was not much difference in weight loss between supplementers and nonsupplementers, there was a huge difference in body fat percentage. The CLA-supplementers dropped from 21.3 percent (average body fat) to an average of 17 percent. While it might not sound like much, a reduction of a few points in body fat percentage can make a huge difference in how lean and firm you look. The people taking CLA lost mostly body fat—the ideal situation in any trim-down program.

If you're already overweight, CLA banishes pounds too, according to a recent study published in the *Journal of Nutrition*. Sixty overweight people randomly took either a placebo or CLA for twelve weeks. The CLA dosage ranged from 1.7 grams to 6.8 grams daily. By the end of the experimental period, those who supplemented with 3.4 grams of CLA daily had dissolved their body fat by six pounds, on average. The researchers concluded that supplementing with 3.4 grams a day is enough to pare down pounds, plus manage your weight.

Another study found that dieters who stopped dieting, but continued to take CLA, were more likely to gain body-firming muscle afterward, rather than ugly fat pounds. This finding hints that CLA may be a great supplement for postdieting maintenance.

One thing to keep in mind: Don't watch for lost pounds on your scale if you're taking CLA. The research cited above clearly points to the fact that CLA gets rid of fat but enhances muscle. Because muscle weighs more than fat, the best way to see the effects of CLA is by checking the notches on your belt, rather than by weighing yourself on a scale. Scales simply don't give the best picture of whether you're tubby or toned, especially if you're supplementing with CLA.

CLA is widely promoted as a fat-burning, energy-boosting agent and is included as a primary ingredient in many weight-loss supplements now on health-food-store shelves. CLA does not require a prescription.

Fights Cardiovascular Disease

Cardiovascular disease is among the most dreaded of all health problems—and for good reason. It is the number one killer of adults in the United States.

Now some astonishingly good news: In addition to diet, exercise, and other healthy lifestyle practices, one way to escape this killer may be supplementation with CLA. That's because, in experimental animals, CLA thwarts the formation of plaque, the fatty deposits in the lining of the artery walls that lead to atherosclerosis.

What's more, animals fed CLA have significantly reduced levels of low-density cholesterol, very-low-density cholesterol, and triglycerides (three nasty conspirators in heart disease).

Further, in an experiment with human blood, CLA blocked a potentially dangerous process called *platelet aggregation,* in which tiny clotting elements in the blood called platelets tend to stick together when they're not supposed to. Clots are apt to form, contributing to heart attack and stroke. CLA may thus help protect against heart disease, but further studies are needed to confirm this benefit.

Protects Against Cancer

Another of the most dreaded diseases known to man is also the second leading cause of death in the United States: cancer. More than 1,500 Americans die of cancer each day, according to the American Cancer Society. Mounds of research with animals reveal that CLA protects against breast cancer, discourages the growth of skin tumors, and shrinks cancerous prostate tumors.

CLA's cancer-fighting properties were discovered in a rather serendipitous way. While investigating carcinogens that occur in grilled meats, University of Wisconsin researchers found that CLA blocked the formation of cancer-causing substances. This amazing finding led to more intensive research on CLA's potential as a cancer-fighter. Many animal studies have since found that it suppresses mammary cancer and skin cancer.

Published in 1996, a large-scale study conducted by Finland's National Public Health Institute produced compelling evidence of CLA's anticancer benefit in humans. Women who drank milk regularly for twenty-five years slashed their odds of getting breast cancer by 50 percent, compared to nonmilk-drinking women. The investigators zeroed in on CLA as the likely agent for the protective effect, since the fatty acid is highly concentrated in milk fat.

A word of advice: There's no CLA in fat-free milk, so many medical experts are recommending that women switch to low-fat milk (which contains CLA) to get possible protection against breast cancer.

What's more, numerous studies have found that CLA is toxic to human breast cancer cells in lab dishes, and slows their growth. And, just-completed human studies in Finland and France indicate that CLA intake is associated with a reduced risk of breast cancer and its recurrence. Moreover, tests conducted with human cancer cells grown in cell cultures show that CLA also inhibits the growth of melanoma, colon cancer, and lung cancer.

Animal research reveals that CLA may also help prevent and reverse a wasting disease called *cachexia,* which occurs when the body burns up muscle to obtain energy for fighting diseases such as cancer. Cachexia compromises the quality of life and long-term survival of cancer patients.

The big question: Just how does CLA put up such a powerful shield against cancer?

Scientists believe that CLA may enhance immunity— in three possible ways. One is by acting as an antioxidant that fights disease-causing free radicals and thus fortifies cellular defenses. Second, CLA appears to reduce the formation of a potentially harmful type of prostaglandin that suppresses T-cells, which identify and destroy cancer cells. This not-so-friendly prostaglandin also shuts down the production of interleukin-2, an immune agent required by T-cells for growth. In other words, CLA bolsters your immune system by making sure immune cells can do their job of killing off cancer cells, without inference from bad prostaglandins. A third theory holds that grazing cows extract anticancer compounds from the pasture vegetables they eat and transfer them to milk. There may be yet-to-be discovered mechanisms at work too, since CLA is made up of different active compounds that may produce different effects.

Defeats Diabetes

Some 2,200 Americans are diagnosed every day with diabetes. Though treatable, diabetes is the seventh leading cause of death in the United States, and nearly 16 million people have it, according to statistics from the American Diabetes Association. Treatment is multifaceted and includes diet, exercise, oral medication, and insulin therapy (depending on what type of diabetes you have).

Emerging new evidence indicates that CLA may be an effective natural therapy for diabetes as well. One study involving prediabetic rats found that CLA improved glucose tolerance (the ability to transport blood glucose into cells for use by the body) and normalized too-high levels of glucose in the blood. The researchers noted that CLA might turn out to be an important therapy for the prevention and treatment of type 2 diabetes, the most common form of the disease.

In a clinical trial, people with poorly controlled diabetes took 3 grams of CLA daily for twelve weeks and were able to bring their blood sugar closer to normal range. In addition, they slashed their triglycerides levels in half. (High triglycerides are frequently diagnosed in people with diabetes and represent a risk for heart disease.)

Outmaneuvers Osteoporosis

Osteoporosis is the most common human bone disease, with 25 million sufferers in the United States alone. In women, bone loss can start as early as ages thirty to thirty-five at the rate of 0.5 to 1 percent a year. In the first three to five years following menopause, this can accelerate to 3 to 7 percent a year, making it possible to lose 9 to 35 percent of bone mass. By age seventy, some women may lose up to 70 percent of their bone mass.

One of the many factors that spells trouble for bones is

prostaglandin E2 (PGE2), one of the so-called bad prostaglandins. Small amounts of PGE2 assist in bone formation, but too much PGE2 inhibits bone growth and has been linked to osteoporosis and arthritis. If you overindulge in omega-6 fats (found in vegetable oils, processed foods, and fast foods), your body steps up its production of PGE2. In studies with rats given CLA, the CLA increased the rate of bone formation while arresting the production of PGE2.

As for human studies, researchers at the University of Memphis investigated the effects of CLA supplementation during weight training on bone mineral (the calcium phosphate in bones) and on certain immune factors. For twenty-eight days, the subjects (twenty-three experienced male weight trainers) took 6 grams a day of CLA, or 9 grams a day of an olive oil placebo. By the end of the experimental period, bone mineral content had increased in the CLA-supplementers; their immune status also improved.

Other than the studies described in this chapter, there has not been much research into CLA and osteoporosis. But stay tuned: Current knowledge about CLA suggests that this supplement represents an avenue of bone research clearly worth pursuing.

SUPPLEMENTING WITH CLA

From the looks of the research, supplementing with CLA may keep you from prematurely going to your grave. With that possibility in mind, how much should you take?

Because most of the research on CLA has been conducted with animals, the appropriate dosage range for people is unknown. Generally, though, the dosage on CLA supplements ranges from 2 to 4 grams daily. Health care practitioners recommend that you take your CLA supplements with food.

Since CLA is so prevalent in food, can you get by with eating dietary sources?

Not really. There's only about 0.14 grams in a 3-ounce hamburger, 0.04 in a glass of whole milk, and 0.03 grams in an ounce of cheese. So gobbling hunks of cheese or swilling gallons of whole milk is not a good way to obtain CLA from the diet, since high-fat foods eaten in excess contribute to heart disease and other serious illnesses.

Although CLA is found in beef, lamb, and dairy products, changes in cattle feed, along with the public's avoidance of fat-rich diets, may mean that Americans are getting 65 percent less CLA than in the past, according to CLA experts. Vegetarians get even less.

Still, taking 3 grams a day is about twenty to forty times the amount you normally get from food if you eat animal products.

Postscript: There appear to be no reported side effects to supplementing with CLA, probably due to the limited research that has been conducted thus far in humans. However, one human trial found that three months of CLA supplementation (4.2 grams daily) increased lipid peroxidation, a harmful cascade of events in which free radicals attack the lipid-rich membranes of cells.

Table 10

IS LECITHIN A FAT-BURNING FAT TOO?

One of the oldest "fat-burning" fats around is lecithin, a phospholipid found in cells and nerve membranes; in egg yolk, soybeans, and corn; and as an essential constituent of animal and vegetable cells. Lecithin helps process cholesterol in the body. It is loaded with the B-vitamin choline, which prevents fat from building up in the liver and shuttles fat into cells to be burned for energy.

Being so high in choline, lecithin has been dubbed a fat burner and is available supplementally in capsules, granules, and liquid form. But there's no proof that it helps you burn fat. Technically, lecithin is a fat, and like a fat, it provides 9 calories per gram, or about 250 calories per ounce. In fact, research shows that a side effect of supplementing with high doses of lecithin is weight gain.

TEN

MCT Oil:
The Dieter's Fat

It's a dieter's dream: a fat that melts fat.

Does such a fat exist? You bet. Meet medium-chain triglyceride (MCT) oil, a special type of dietary fat that was first formulated in the 1950s by the pharmaceutical industry for patients who had trouble digesting regular fats. Since then, MCT oil has been used therapeutically to treat fat malabsorption, cystic fibrosis, and obesity. In the last fifteen years, it has been employed effectively as a sports supplement and as a nutritional supplement that aids in weight loss and helps boost energy.

MCT oil is processed mainly from coconut oil but does not seem to have any of the adverse side effects associated with tropical oils, such as elevated LDL cholesterol. It occurs naturally in many of the foods we eat and is quite plentiful in breast milk.

MCT oil is no ordinary fat. Although it tastes much like regular salad oil, that's where the similarities end. At the molecular level, MCT oil is structured very differently from conventional oils and thus has some unique properties.

Conventional fats are made up of long carbon chains, with sixteen or more carbon atoms strung together. MCT oil, on the other hand, has a much shorter carbon chain of only six to twelve carbon atoms—hence its name, medium-chain triglyceride. Because of its shorter chain, MCT oil is metabolized much more quickly than fatty acids from regular oils or fats.

Also, unlike other fats, medium-chain fats are more water soluble. They can be absorbed more easily through the intestinal wall, requiring fewer enzymes or bile salts. In the intestines, MCT oil is broken down into fatty fragments, which combine with a water-soluble protein in the blood. From there, MCTs go right into the bloodstream and are transported to the liver, where, inside the cells, they are rapidly oxidized or burned up.

Basically, very little of this remarkable fat leaves the liver; therefore, MCTs rarely end up being stored as body fat—a scenario does not occur with conventional fats. So by using MCT oil, you can have your fat and eat it too, because it is burned immediately for energy and therefore is not stored as body fat like conventional fats and oils are.

Anyone who is interested in weight control or exercise performance should explore the merits of supplementing with MCT oil. Here is a closer look at what this supplement can do for you.

Stimulates Thermogenesis

MCT oil is burned up so quickly that its calories are turned into body heat—a process known as *thermogenesis,* which boosts your metabolism—your body's food-to-fuel process. The higher your metabolism, the more calories your body burns.

Several studies in animals and humans have tested MCT oil's thermogenic effect. An often-cited study that looked into this effect was published in the journal *Metabolism* in 1989. To determine whether MCT oil affected thermogenesis differently from regular fats, ten men (ages twenty-two to forty-four) were fed with liquid diets containing 40 percent of fat as either MCTs or regular fats. After five days on this diet, thermogenesis increased significantly in the men who consumed MCTs—but remained unchanged in the men who ate regular fats. The researchers concluded that MCT oil stimulated thermogenesis to a greater degree than an equivalent amount of conventional fat did. They also noted that MCT oil was less likely to be stored, in contrast to conventional fats.

Revs Up Metabolism

Have you ever felt like you're losing fat at a snail's pace, or not at all?

Perhaps your metabolism has slowed down and needs a nudge. This often happens in response to low-calorie dieting. In fact, research shows that your metabolic rate drops considerably during a period of caloric restriction. With a sluggish metabolism, your body can't burn calories efficiently, and it's difficult to pare pounds, even though you're on a diet.

Try adding MCT oil to your food to counter this effect. Researchers in Czechoslovakia discovered that when obese patients, who were following a low-calorie diet, supplemented with MCT oil (1 tablespoon daily), their metabolic rate stayed elevated. Thus, incorporating MCT oil into your weight-loss diet may help prevent those frustrating plateaus that dieters so often hit.

Another study corroborates this benefit. In an experiment involving seven healthy men at the University of Rochester, researchers tested whether a single meal of MCTs would increase the metabolic rate more than long-chain fat meal would. The men ate test meals containing 48 grams of MCT oil or 45 grams of corn oil, given in random order on separate days.

Metabolic rate increased 12 percent over six hours after the men ate the MCT meals but increased only 4 percent after corn oil was consumed. What's more, concentrations of fats in plasma (the liquid portion of blood) were elevated 68 percent after the corn oil meal, but did not change after the MCT meal. These findings led the researchers to speculate that replacing conventional oils with MCTs over a long period of time might be beneficial in weight loss.

Burns Fat

Because MCT oil revs up your metabolism, you can potentially burn more fat. In a single-blind, randomized, crossover study, twenty healthy men ingested a single dose of either 71 grams of MCT oil or canola oil. Blood samples were taken prior to the dosing, then at one-hour intervals over five hours following supplementation. Triglycerides, or blood fats, actually decreased 15 percent as a result of taking MCT oil, whereas fats increased 47 percent with canola oil. These findings are quite remarkable: MCT oil burns up and reduces fatty substances in the body. The ramifications of this finding are important for anyone who wants to achieve and maintain a trim physique.

Burns Calories

The best way to do away with stored body fat is to consume fewer calories than your body needs to meet its physical and metabolic demands. So to lose fat, you must create a calorie deficit, either by eating less, exercising more, or both. Now, according to a recent scientific study, there's another way to get that deficit—without sweating or depriving yourself—but by supplementing with MCT oil.

When eight healthy men at the University of Geneva took just 1 to 2 tablespoons of MCT oil as part of their normal diet, their daily caloric expenditure increased by 5 percent! On average, they burned 113 extra calories a day.

What does this mean to you? Suppose, for example, you're eating roughly 2,000 calories a day, with part of those calories coming from MCT oil. You'd effortlessly spend an additional 100 calories a day—the equivalent of walking for thirty minutes at a moderate pace. You'd burn extra calories, without any extra effort!

Enhances Muscle

A healthy goal of any fat-loss program is to preserve as much muscle tissue as possible. The more muscle you have, the better your body can burn fat. This is because muscle is the body's most metabolically active tissue. It burns calories, even at rest. Fat tissue is not as active.

Unfortunately, far too many diets overrestrict calories. Severe caloric restriction forces the body to start cannibalizing its own precious muscle tissue (including heart tissue) for energy.

You can guard your muscle by following a calorie-

adequate diet, sticking to an exercise program that includes strength training—and supplementing with MCT
oil. In a study at Calgary University in Alberta, Canada,
healthy adults were placed on a low-carbohydrate diet
supplemented with MCT oil. The researchers measured
the use of fat and protein in the subjects' bodies and found
that there was an increase in body fat burned and a decrease in muscle protein used for energy. In other words,
MCTs helped burn fat and, at the same time, preserved
lean muscle by preventing its breakdown.

Increases Endurance

Exercise is an important way to encourage fat loss. The
harder and longer you exercise, the more fat you can burn.
But often it's tough to exercise all-out, and one reason is
low energy. That's where MCT oil can help.

First, it provides twice the energy of protein and carbohydrate (8.3 calories per gram versus 4 calories per
gram for carbohydrates and protein) and is absorbed into
the bloodstream as rapidly as glucose, the cellular fuel
made available from the breakdown of carbohydrates.

Second, MCT oil is preferentially used as fuel for energy, instead of being stored by the body. Medium-chain
fatty acid fragments can diffuse into the cell very quickly,
where they are burned immediately for energy—at the
same time as glucose. The ability of MCTs to enter the
cells in this manner has a glucose-sparing effect, meaning
that glucose and its stored counterpart, muscle glycogen,
last longer without being depleted. The longer glycogen
reserves last, the more energy you have for activities and
fat-burning exercise.

To boost your endurance during exercise, take MCT oil
with a carbohydrate source such as a sports drink. At the

University of Capetown Medical School in South Africa, researchers mixed 86 grams of MCT oil (nearly 3 tablespoons) with two liters of 10-percent glucose drink to see what effect it would have on the performance of six endurance-trained cyclists. The cyclists drank a beverage consisting of glucose alone, glucose plus MCT oil, or MCT oil alone. In the laboratory, they pedaled at moderate intensity for about two hours and then completed a higher-intensity time trial. They performed this cycling bout on three separate occasions so that each cyclist used each type of drink once. The cyclists sipped the drink every ten minutes. Performance improved the most when the cyclists supplemented with the MCT/glucose mixture. The researchers did some further biochemical tests on the cyclists and confirmed that the combination spared glycogen while making fat more accessible for fuel.

USING MCT OIL IN A FAT-LOSS DIET

*If you want to jump-start your weight-loss efforts, re*place some of the carbohydrates in your diet with MCT oil. Carbohydrates such as rice, cereal, pasta, breads, fruits, potatoes, and sweet potatoes offer a mother lode of vital nutrients. But too much carbohydrate in your diet can be fat-forming, particularly if you're not very active. A carbohydrate overload triggers a surge of the hormone insulin into your bloodstream. Insulin activates fat cell enzymes that move fat from the bloodstream into fat cells for storage, and this action spells extra weight for many of us.

When you reduce your intake of carbohydrates, you suppress the release of insulin. Low insulin stimulates the release of another hormone, glucagon. As glucagon goes to work, it signals the body to start burning fat for energy.

Reducing carbohydrate intake to lose weight has long been the basis of many diets. And for good reason—it works. But there are penalties. Carbohydrate is your body's leading nutrient fuel. During digestion, carbohydrate is broken down into glucose. Glucose circulates in the blood to be used for energy. If your muscles are deprived of glucose, your physical power suffers. You're low on gas and feel it. It becomes tough to stick to your eating program, and another attempt to lose weight could bite the dust.

But MCT oil can come to the rescue. You can still apply the low-carbohydrate dieting strategy, but without the corresponding loss of energy! Remember: MCT oil is burned in the body like a carbohydrate and spares glucose fuel for an energy-boosting effect.

Thus, by supplementing with MCT oil, you have a pure energy source to help prevent diet-induced fatigue. At the same time, MCT oil keeps your metabolism high, and a high metabolism is conducive to losing body fat.

How, then, should you plan your weight-loss diet to take advantage of MCT oil's powers? Here are some guidelines that explain how to substitute MCT oil for high-starch carbohydrate foods to facilitate fat-burning:

- Design a diet with the following percentages of nutrients: 20 to 25 percent protein, 40 to 50 percent carbohydrates, and the rest from fat, including MCT oil. Along with the restriction of carbohydrates, the higher percentage of protein in the diet helps control hormones too (less insulin, more glucagon) in favor of fat loss.

- Eat higher-starch carbohydrate foods such as cereals,

whole grains, potatoes, legumes, bread, pasta, or fruit only at breakfast, your midmorning snack, and lunch to adequately fuel your daily activities. (For carbohydrates, stick to natural ones such as potatoes and whole grains. Natural carbohydrates are used more efficiently by the body than their processed counterparts—breads and pastas, for example—because they are preferentially stored as glycogen, rather than as fat, if not used first for energy.)

* Do not eat any higher-starch carbohydrates after lunch.

* Use MCT oil (up to a tablespoon), taken with some nonstarchy vegetables for an afternoon snack. Have some additional MCT oil as salad dressing at dinner. Used this way, MCT oil moves your body into a fat-burning mode and helps speed up your metabolism.

* Stay on a diet plan like this no more than two weeks at a time.

SUPPLEMENTING WITH MCT OIL

MCT oil should always be taken with food and can be drizzled over vegetables or made into salad dressings (see the recipes in chapter 12). You can also cook or bake with MCT oil just as you would with any other vegetable oil. Keep the heat at 350 degrees or lower, however, because MCT oil smokes at high temperatures. Don't store MCT oil in anything other than a glass container. It tends to soften containers made of certain types of plastic.

Gradually introduce MCT oil into your diet at the rate of a few teaspoons a day until you are eating two to three tablespoons a day. MCT oil contains 120 calories per tablespoon. This supplement is so rapidly absorbed that it tends to cause stomach cramping if too much is taken at one time or on an empty stomach.

Make sure you purchase pure MCT oil, not a product that's diluted. How can you tell? A good rule of thumb is that any MCT oil product that comes flavored is not the pure stuff. Read the label to see whether the product is cut with flavorings or other fillers.

SAFETY CONSIDERATIONS

MCT oil is generally safe for most people, except those with preexisting medical conditions. The supplement is not advised if you have a fatty liver or cirrhosis, because the fat is channeled directly into an already poorly working liver. Nor should you use MCT oil if you suffer from a chronic pulmonary disease such as emphysema or asthma, because it results in greater production of carbon dioxide—a side effect that can further complicate breathing. If you are diabetic, avoid MCT oil too, because it promotes the production of ketones, by-products of fat-burning that are dangerous to people with this disease.

Worth mentioning too: Extensive studies with animals have shown that MCTs do not have the potential to be carcinogenic.

MCT oil does not supply essential fatty acids, so make sure you're eating at least 2 teaspoons of such fats daily. Never substitute MCT oil entirely for essential fats in your diet, or else you'll risk an essential fatty acid deficiency.

PART V.

Designing a Fat-Healthy Diet

ELEVEN

A Smart-Fat Strategy

Without question, few nutrition topics have stirred up so much confusion as that of dietary fat. With conflicting recommendations on which fats to eat and which fats to avoid, it's easy to get overwhelmed. But don't despair. The first step is to give some thought to your personal health situation and decide what's best for you. For example: Do you have high cholesterol? Do you need to lose weight? Are you suffering from a health problem that might be treated with a fat supplement?

Once you've answered these questions, begin revamping your nutrition program to control both the amount and the type of fat you eat. There are some fats you'll want to include routinely in your diet, others you'll want to avoid, and still others you may want to take therapeutically, like medicine, on a temporary basis.

In this chapter there are several health scenarios. See where you fit in and note the recommendations. Once you've identified your niche, follow the recommendations, but tweak them where necessary. With nutrition, the key is to adopt healthy eating habits but to customize them to your lifestyle.

GENERAL GOOD FAT GUIDELINES FOR EVERYONE

By commandeering dietary fat—the type and the amount—you can stay healthy and delay or even prevent many life-threatening diseases. To help, the American Heart Association has developed dietary guidelines designed to promote good health and prevent disease. These guidelines are an excellent reference for deciding how much fat you need in your diet. Although mentioned elsewhere in this book, they bear repeating:

• Saturated fat should be held to 7 to 10 percent of your total calories (the number of calories you need to achieve and maintain a healthy body weight).

• Polyunsaturated fat intake should be up to 10 percent of your total calories.

• Monounsaturated fat should compose up to 15 percent of your total calories.

• Total fat intake should be no more than 30 percent of your total calories (600 calories a day based on a 2,000-calories-a-day diet). This guideline applies to total calories eaten over several days, such as a week.

If you're a math lover, you can calculate your own daily fat intake by using the following formulas:

Total fat: Total calories per day ×.30 = daily fat calories

Daily fat calories / 9 = _____ daily fat grams

(For example: 1,200 calories ×.30 = 360 daily fat calories; 360 daily fat calories / 9 = 40 daily fat grams)

Saturated fatty acids (SFA): Total calories per day ×.07 = daily SFA calories

Daily SFA calories / 9 = daily SFA grams

(For example: 1,200 calories ×.07 = 84 daily SFA calories; 84 daily SFA calories / 9 = 9 daily SFA grams)

Polyunsaturated fatty acids (PUFA): Total calories ×.10 = daily PUFA calories

Daily PUFA calories / 9 = daily PUFA grams

(For example: 1,200 calories ×.10 = 100 daily PUFA calories; 100 daily PUFA calories / 9 = 13 daily PUFA grams)

Monounsaturated fatty acids (MUFA): Total calories ×.15 = daily MUFA calories

Daily MUFA calories / 9 = daily MUFA grams

(For example: 1,200 calories ×.15 = 100 daily MUFA calories; 100 daily MUFA calories / 9 = 20 daily MUFA grams)

Table 11 shows how these recommendations and calculations translate into actual grams of fat.

Table 11

GRAMS OF FAT AND CALORIC LEVELS

Calorie Level	Saturated Fats (grams)	Polyunsaturated Fats (grams)	Monounsaturated Fats (grams)	Total Fats (grams)
1,200	9	13	20	40 or less
1,500	12	16	25	50 or less
1,800	14	20	30	60 or less
2,000	16	22	33	67 or less
2,200	17	24	36	73 or less
2,500	19	28	42	83 or less
3,000	23	33	50	100 or less

Once you've calculated your own dietary allowance for total fat and saturated fat, be sure to read food labels for the fat content per serving. The grams of fat are listed under *nutrition facts* on any food package that provides a nutrition label.

Another way to monitor your fat intake is by limiting the majority of foods in your diet to those that have only 30 percent or less of their calories from fat. By using the information on the nutrition label, you can easily determine if a food meets this criterion. Use the following formula to find percentage of calories from fat:

Percent calories from fat = Calories of fat per serving / total calories per serving × 100

Suppose an item of food has 36 fat calories in a serving, and the total calories per serving are 220. Here's an example using that label information:

36 fat calories/220 calories per serving × 100 = 16%
of calories from fat

In addition to controlling the amount of fat you eat, you must make good fat choices. Some of this information has been covered in previous chapters, but here's a quick summary for review:

Increase your intake of omega-3 fatty acids.

Eat cold-water fish two to three times a week. Fish servings should be at least 3 ounces—about the size of a deck of cards. In addition, use flaxseed in recipes and meals, or eat a tablespoon of flaxseed oil each day. Flaxseed is the richest plant source of alpha-linolenic acid, an omega-3 fatty acid.

Put more monounsaturated acids in your diet.

Use extra-virgin olive oil in salad dressings, for bread dipping, or for cooking. Canola oil is another fat high in monosaturated fats that makes an excellent oil for cooking or baking. In addition, use avocados in salads; they are chock-full of healthy monounsaturated fats. Also loaded with these good fats are nuts. Sprinkle them on cereal, yogurt, salads, and other foods.

Cut back on omega-6 fats.

These include vegetable oils such as corn, cottonseed, safflower seed, sunflower seed, and soybean oils—and products like margarines that are made from them. For margarines, opt for spreads made with canola oil instead.

Processed foods are also high in omega-6 fats and should thus be limited in your diet.

Curtail your saturated fats.

These are found mostly in fatty cuts of meat, poultry skin, whole and 2-percent milk, cheese, butter, many ice creams, and coconut oil. Here are some easy ways to control your intake of saturated fats:

- Choose lean cuts of good- or choice-grade meat like round, sirloin, and flank, and eat portions that are no larger than the palm of your hand. Chicken, turkey, and fish are always leaner meat choices, or substitute fish a couple of times during the week.

- When preparing and eating meats, make sure to trim all visible fat and skin, and use cooking racks to bake, broil, grill, steam, or microwave, to avoid melting the fat back into the meat.

- When eating lunch meats, select low-fat or fat-free chicken or turkey breast, rather than high-fat bologna or salami.

- Choose low-fat or skimmed products rather than whole milk, and include them two to three times each day.

- Eat reduced-fat or fat-free cheese.

Eliminate or limit trans-fats.

Found in processed foods and fast foods, these fats are the "baddest" of the bad, linked to heart disease and many other life-threatening illnesses. Check the labels of foods and select products without partially hydrogenated oils in the list of ingredients. Switch to margarines that are trans-free. Also, nix the fried foods at restaurants. Chances are, they're prepared in oils full of trans-fats.

GUIDELINES FOR HIGH CHOLESTEROL

To bring your cholesterol down, you need to reduce your intake of saturated fat and dietary cholesterol. The American Heart Association recommends that you:

- Restrict your fat intake to 30 percent of your total calories. Less than 7 percent of your total calories should come from saturated fats and trans-fats.

- Limit your daily intake of dietary cholesterol to less than 200 milligrams.

- Select nonfat dairy products.

- Eat no more than 6 ounces a day of lean meat, fish, or skinless poultry.

- Restrict your use of fats and oils to five to eight servings a day. (For examples of servings, see Box 12.)

- Eat five or more daily servings of fruits and vegetables, and six or more servings of grains—bread, cereal, or rice, for example.

Beyond these recommendations, there are others measures worth taking. For example, two or three times a day, try substituting butter and margarine with cholesterol-lowering spreads such as Benecol or Take Control. Both have been clinically proven to reduce total cholesterol and LDL cholesterol.

In addition, eat flaxseed as a regular part of your diet,

supplement with evening primrose oil (3 to 4 grams a day), and use olive oil in your cooking as part of your allowable daily fat portion.

Also, be careful to not overindulge on sugary foods. Research has shown that sugar may be a risk factor for heart disease, possibly because it generates very-low-density lipoprotein (VLDL) cholesterol and triglycerides. Both are harmful to the heart. Thus, avoid products listing more than 5 grams of sugar per serving on the label. If the specific amount of sugar is unlisted, shun products with sugar listed as one of the first four ingredients on the label. Sugar goes by various other names too: sucrose, dextrose, maltose, lactose, maltodextrin, corn syrup, to name just a few.

In addition to dietary measures, begin a regular exercise program—and stick with it. Exercising can lower your cholesterol by about 9 percent and raise your HDL cholesterol by 5 to 15 percent. The key is to do at least thirty minutes of exercise most days of the week.

If your cholesterol doesn't drop with diet and exercise, consult your physician. You may need a cholesterol-lowering medication.

GUIDELINES FOR HIGH TRIGLYCERIDES

Triglycerides are the chemical form in which fat exists in food, as well as in body fat. They're also present in blood plasma, and together with cholesterol, form the lipids in your blood.

High blood triglycerides are most often associated with heart disease and may be a consequence of type 2 diabetes. Table 13 lists the various measurements for triglycerides.

Several factors can elevate your triglyceride levels:

Table 12

CONTROLLING CHOLESTEROL:
SERVINGS AND SELECTIONS FOR FATS AND OILS

Servings per day	Serving Size
5 to 8 servings	1 tsp. vegetable oil or regular margarine 2 tsp. diet margarine 1 tbsp. salad dressing 2 tsp. mayonnaise or peanut butter 3 tsp. seeds or nuts 1/8 medium avocado 10 small or 5 large olives
Choose from:	Vegetable oils or margarines with no more than 2 grams of saturated fat per tablespoon: canola, corn, olive, safflower, sesame, soybean, sunflower, and walnut; and almond, avocado, and hazelnut monounsaturated oils. For margarines, choose those that contain liquid vegetable oil as the first ingredient. For mayonnaise and salad dressing, select those with no more than 1 gram of saturated fat per tablespoon.

Source: American Heart Association.

drinking alcohol, taking estrogen, and poorly controlling your diabetes. Higher-carbohydrate diets tend to increase triglycerides too. So does eating too much high-fructose corn syrup, a refined version of fructose made from corn and found in many processed foods and beverages.

Reducing your triglycerides requires a lifestyle fix in which your goals are to lose weight (if you're overweight), reduce the cholesterol and saturated fat in your diet, avoid or limit alcohol consumption, and become more active.

Table 13

TRIGLYCERIDE READINGS

Normal triglycerides	Less than 200 mg/dl
Borderline-high triglycerides	200 to 400 mg/dl
High triglycerides	400 to 1,000 mg/dl
Very high triglycerides	Greater than 1,000 mg/dl

Source: American Heart Association

Also urged by medical experts is substituting monounsaturated fats and polyunsaturated fats for saturated fats. With this approach, 40 percent of your total daily calories should come from fat. However, half of that fat should come from monounsaturated fats, which have been shown in research to lower triglyceride levels. A higher monounsaturated fat diet might include olive oil or canola oil as part of your daily diet. When you increase your calories from fat, be careful not to increase your total calories, particularly if you're trying to watch your weight. In addition, reduce your intake of carbohydrates because they elevate triglycerides and decrease HDL cholesterol.

Fat supplements that may help regulate triglycerides include perilla oil and DHA.

GUIDELINES FOR HIGH BLOOD PRESSURE

*A low-fat diet designed to control cholesterol is also ben*eficial for reducing high blood pressure (hypertension), particularly if it includes plentiful amounts of fruits, vegetables, whole grains, and low-fat dairy products. This type of diet is rich in nutrients such as calcium, potassium, and magnesium, all of which help normalize blood pressure.

One mineral that should be restricted, however, is sodium, found in table salt. Too much salt in the body tends to narrow the diameter of blood vessels. When this happens, the heart has to work harder to pump the same amount of blood, and blood pressure soars as a result. Excessive salt also makes the body retain too much water, and this may cause a rise in blood pressure.

If you suffer from high blood pressure, do not add salt to your food and avoid salty foods such as snack food, smoked meats, pickled foods, cheese and cheese products, fast foods, and canned foods. If you miss the taste of salt on foods, try a salt substitute or experiment with various herbs and spices when cooking.

Healthy fats that may help drive blood pressure down include fish oil supplements (and fish), borage oil, black currant oil, and olive oil.

Losing weight helps normalize blood pressure too. On average, you can cut your blood pressure by several points by losing weight through diet and exercise.

Another way to reduce high blood pressure is with aerobic exercise, such as walking, jogging, running, swimming, bicycling, and so forth. Most studies of hypertensive people show that a reduction can occur with as little as three exercise sessions a week for thirty to sixty minutes each time.

If your blood pressure can't be controlled by lifestyle changes, you'll probably need to take medication prescribed by your doctor.

GUIDELINES FOR WEIGHT LOSS

Being overweight, defined as 20 percent or more above your ideal weight, puts you in harm's way of numerous life-threatening diseases. Among them: heart problems (overweight increases LDL cholesterol and lowers HDL cholesterol), stroke, high blood pressure, and diabetes.

Without question, it can be challenging to lose weight, especially if you're way off the ideal. But it's not impossible either.

The first step is to eat fewer calories than your body uses each day. To lose a pound of body fat, you have to create a 3,500-calorie deficit, either by eating less, exercising more, or both. By cutting your total calorie intake by 500 calories each day, for example, you should be able to lose one pound a week (500 calories × 7 days)—a safe rate of weight loss. If you add exercise to this equation and burn any extra calories, your fat loss will be even greater. An hour of exercise, for example, can burn up anywhere from 250 to 500 calories.

Your weight-loss diet should be as low in fat as possible, since reducing dietary fat is one of the best ways to shed pounds. By keeping your total fat intake to 20 percent of total daily calories, you may be able to lose body fat with less restriction in total calories.

In addition, try to curb your intake of fat-forming foods such as sugar, processed foods, and alcohol. By limiting these foods, you'll automatically reduce the number of calories in your diet.

Two fat supplements that may help you lose body fat are conjugated linoleic acid (3 grams daily) and medium-chain triglyceride oil (MCT oil). Try substituting MCT oil for some of your fat calories each day and for a portion of your higher-starch carbohydrates. MCT oil revs up your metabolism to help your body burn energy more efficiently.

In addition to the diet tips, many people have successfully lost weight by following a higher-fat, moderate-protein, and restricted-carbohydrate diet. Generally, these diets work by encouraging your body to switch from burning stored carbohydrate (glycogen) for energy to burning stored body fat. One of the most popular low-carbohydrate diets is the Atkins Diet.

In a study of the diet conducted at the Durham VA Medical Center in North Carolina, mildly obese people lost about twenty-one pounds in four months on the diet. What's more, they showed a 6.1 percent drop in cholesterol, a 40-percent decline in triglycerides, and an increase in HDL cholesterol by about 7 percent.

The diet restricted carbohydrate intake to less than 20 grams daily and included vitamin supplements, fish oil supplements, and twenty minutes of exercise at least three times a week.

Not all diets work equally well for everyone. You should choose a weight-loss diet that fits your food preferences and lifestyle. Further, it should be a diet you're willing to stick with for the long haul, in order to lose the required amount of weight.

GUIDELINES FOR DIABETES

Diabetes is a complex disease, requiring treatment that involves diet, exercise, lifestyle changes, and, for many people, injectable insulin or oral diabetes drugs. Generally, the recommended diet is one similar to that for high cholesterol: a low-saturated fat, low-cholesterol, high-fiber diet. In addition, a number of good fats may be therapeutically beneficial for treating diabetes: flaxseeds and flaxseed oil, black currant oil, evening primrose oil, and, possibly, DHA. Fish oil supplements are generally not recommended if you have diabetes. Rely on fish to get your dose of its essential fatty acids.

High triglycerides tend to occur simultaneously with high LDLs and low HDLs. If your diabetes is complicated by high triglycerides (greater than 250 mg/dl), the American Diabetes Association suggests that you try a higher-fat diet in which 40 percent of your total daily calories is derived from fat. However, half of your fat should come from monounsaturated fats, which have been shown in research to lower triglyceride levels.

GUIDELINES FOR ARTHRITIS

*Arthritis, a serious and potentially crippling disease, af*fects millions of people worldwide. It attacks the joints as well as the muscle and connective tissues surrounding them. There are more than 100 different forms of arthritis. The two most common are osteoarthritis, caused by wear and tear on the joints, and rheumatoid arthritis, an autoimmune disease in which the body's immune system attacks itself.

To some extent, supplements can play a role in treating arthritis. Omega-3 fatty acids such as fish oil and flaxseed oil are helpful in relieving symptoms. So are GLA-rich supplements such as borage oil, black currant oil, and evening primrose oil. Another good move is to reduce your intake of saturated fat such as red meat, dairy products (whole milk, 2-percent milk, ice cream, butter, cheese, cream), margarine, shortening, lard, cocoa butter, and fried foods. The less saturated fat you eat, the better omega-3 fats can work their healing magic.

THERAPEUTIC USE OF ESSENTIAL FATTY ACID SUPPLEMENTS

The essential fatty acid supplements discussed in this book are simply nutrients, extracted from food or plants, that have a much gentler effect on the body than do prescription drugs. That being so, you may want to take certain supplements from time to time, on a therapeutic basis, to help alleviate symptoms or coax your body to heal naturally. In certain circumstances—say a migraine or menstrual pain—it's usually wise to try the gentler agent first, before resorting to prescription or over-the-counter drugs. Do so with the okay of your physician or psychiatrist, however, particularly since essential fatty acid supplements contain factors that may thin your blood, which can increase bleeding times.

You may experience some other mild side effects from taking essential fatty acid supplements, including upset stomach, burping, or minor bowel problems such as loose stools. These can minimized by taking the supplement with meals and in divided doses throughout the day.

As fats, essential fatty acid supplements contain calories. Typically, there are about 10 calories in a 1,000-milligram softgel, so you'll need to take this into consideration if you're counting calories.

Many manufacturers make essential fatty acid supplements that contain a blend of various omega-3 and omega-6 fats. These may worth a try to ensure that you get a good balance of the right fats.

The following chart (Table 14) reviews the various disorders that can be treated with essential fatty acid supplements and provides the dosages generally recommended by health care practitioners.

Table 14

TREATING DISEASE WITH ESSENTIAL FATTY ACID SUPPLEMENTS

Disorder/Illness	Supplements	Dosage	Comments
Abnormal clotting	Flaxseed oil Perilla oil	40 grams daily 6 grams daily	Check with your physician because EFA supplements may thin your blood, or interfere with the action of blood-thinning medication.
ARDS	Borage oil	Consult your physician regarding dosage.	Supplementation should support conventional medical treatment under the care of a physician.
Arrhythmias	Fish oil	4 grams daily	Supplementation should support conventional medical treatment under the care of a physician.
Asthma	Perilla oil	6 grams daily	Supplementation should support conventional medical treatment under the care of a physician.
Brain diseases	DHA	100 milligrams daily if you eat fish; 200 milligrams daily if you eat no fish.	Supplementation should support conventional medical treatment under the care of a physician.

Table 14 continued

TREATING DISEASE WITH ESSENTIAL FATTY ACID SUPPLEMENTS

Disorder/Illness	Supplements	Dosage	Comments
Breast pain	Evening primrose oil	6 grams daily	Supplementation often works better than standard drug treatment.
Depression	Fish oil	6 grams daily	Supplementation should support conventional medical treatment under the care of a physician or psychiatrist.
Diabetes	DHA may be helpful, although research is preliminary.	Correct dosage for treating diabetes is unknown.	Take supplements only after consultation with your physician and dietitian.
Diabetic nerve damage	Evening primrose oil	1–4 grams daily	Supplementation should support conventional medical treatment under the care of a physician.
Eczema	Evening primrose oil	1–4 grams daily	One of the best natural treatments available for eczema.
High cholesterol	Evening primrose oil	1–4 grams daily	Should be used in conjunction with a cholesterol-lowering diet that includes reduced intake of saturated fats.

Table 14 continued

TREATING DISEASE WITH ESSENTIAL FATTY ACID SUPPLEMENTS

Disorder/Illness	Supplements	Dosage	Comments
High triglycerides	Fish oil	100 milligrams daily if you eat fish;·200 milligrams daily if you eat no fish.	Should be used in conjunction with a low-fat diet in which 40 percent of fat calories are derived from monounsaturated fats.
	DHA	3 grams daily	
	CLA	Up to 3 grams daily	
	Perilla oil	6 grams daily	
Hypertension	Fish oil	3 grams daily	Supplementation should support conventional medical treatment under the care of a physician. Borage oil should not be taken with anticonvulsants.
	Borage oil	3 grams daily	
Inflammatory bowel disease	Fish oil	3 grams daily	Supplementation should support conventional medical treatment under the care of a physician.
Menstrual disorders	Evening primrose oil	1–4 grams daily	One of the most effective natural treatments for a variety of menstrual problems, including cramps, premenstrual syndrome (PMS), breast pain, and heavy bleeding.

Table 14 continued

TREATING DISEASE WITH ESSENTIAL FATTY ACID SUPPLEMENTS

Disorder/Illness	Supplements	Dosage	Comments
Migraines	Evening primrose oil	1–4 grams daily	Relieves inflammation associated with migraine pain.
Obesity	CLA	3–4 grams daily	Should be used in conjunction with a low-fat, reduced-calorie diet, plus regular exercise.
	MCT oil	1–2 tablespoons daily to replace some of daily fat portion	
Osteoarthritis	Lyprinol (green-lipped–mussel supplement)	210 milligrams daily	Supplementation should support conventional medical treatment under the care of a physician.
Psoriasis	EPA	1.8 grams daily	Supplementation should support conventional medical treatment under the care of a physician.
Rheumatoid arthritis	Black currant oil	525 milligrams daily	Supplementation should support conventional medical treatment under the care of a physician.
	Borage oil	1.4 grams daily	
	Fish oil	3–5 grams daily	

TWELVE

Good Fat Cooking

*There's certainly no better way to start reaping the ben-*efits of good fats than to start cooking with them. Using healthful fats and oils such as MCT oil, flaxseeds and flaxseed oil, olive oil, canola oil, and sesame seeds and sesame oil in recipes is an effortless way to get a healthy dose of essential fats, monounsaturated fats, and other good-for-you fats. With that in mind, here are some recipes that incorporate many of the fats discussed in this book.

MCT OIL RECIPES

Medium-chain triglyceride (MCT oil) is a special type of dietary fat that is metabolized quickly and not easily stored as body fat. It is a useful supplement if you are trying to trim down and get in shape. You can also cook or bake with MCT oil just as you would with any other vegetable oil. Keep the heat at 350 degrees or lower, however, because MCT oil smokes at high temperatures.

The following MCT oil recipes are used with permission from Parrillo Performance, 4690K Interstate Drive, Cincinnati, Ohio 45246, 800-344-3404. This company makes an unflavored MCT oil product called CapTri®.

Fried Chicken

2 cups shredded wheat (crumbled very fine)

¼ cup oat bran

1 tsp. onion powder

½ tsp. garlic powder

½ tsp. barbecue seasoning

½ tsp. coarse black pepper

1 tsp. Mrs. Dash Lemon and Herb seasoning

2 pounds chicken breasts

5 tbsp. MCT oil (unflavored)

Place chicken in medium-sized glass bowl and coat thoroughly with MCT oil. Set aside.

In another bowl, mix all other ingredients for breading. Dip chicken one piece at a time into the breading mixture and toss until well coated.

Heat skillet (moderate heat) with any remaining MCT oil from the chicken dip. Reduce heat to low and cover. Turn chicken breasts occasionally to cook evenly on all sides. Chicken is done when breading is brown and meat is white, juicy and tender. Be careful to not overcook, as this will dry out your chicken and make it tough.

Makes 5 servings.
438 calories per serving; 19 grams of fat per serving.

◆ ◆ ◆

Cod Fillet Italiano

2 lbs. cod fillets

1 cup oatmeal flour

3½ cups chopped tomato, blended in blender

3 tbsp. minced parsley

1 tsp. oregano

¼ tsp. garlic powder

¼ tsp. onion powder

⅛ tsp. pepper

2 tbsp. MCT oil (unflavored)

Preheat oven to 325 degrees. In a small bowl, combine oatmeal flour, parsley, and other seasonings with 1 tbsp. MCT oil. Spread remaining MCT oil in the bottom of a 9-inch baking dish. Spread oatmeal flour mixture evenly over the fillets. Bake for 20 minutes. Remove from oven and pour blended tomatoes over fillets. Bake for an additional 10 to 15 minutes, or until fish flakes when tested with a fork.

Makes 4 servings.
350 calories per serving; 10 grams of fat per serving.

◆ ◆ ◆

Mexican Black Bean and Turkey Salad

3/4 tsp. cumin

3/4 tsp. chili powder

1/8 tsp. salt

1/8 tsp. ground pepper

1 lb. turkey breast, cut into strips

1 cup curly endive

1 cup romaine lettuce

1/2 cup fresh orange segments

1/4 cup chopped red onion

2 1/2 cups black beans, washed and drained

1/2 cup cilantro

1/4 cup lime juice

3 tbsp. MCT oil (unflavored)

Extra MCT oil for cooking

1/8 tsp. salt

1 small garlic clove, chopped

1 tbsp. fresh orange juice

Place cumin, chili powder, salt, and ground pepper in a bag and shake to mix. Add turkey to bag and continue shaking to coat turkey. Let marinate for 1 to 3 hours. Saute turkey in skillet lightly coated with MCT oil until golden brown on the outside.

Mix endive and romaine lettuce with orange segments, onions, black beans, and cilantro. Add turkey.

For dressing, mix lime juice, MCT oil, salt, garlic, and orange juice. Toss with vegetable and turkey mixture.

Makes 5 servings.
485 calories per serving; 12.5 grams of fat per serving.

◆ ◆ ◆

White Chili

2 ½ cups canned white beans

1 quart water

1 quart chicken stock

1 cup chopped onions

3 chopped garlic cloves

½ chopped green chili peppers

2 tsp. cumin

1½ tsp. crushed oregano

1 tsp. coriander

¼ tsp. cloves

¼ tsp. cayenne pepper

1 lb. baked turkey breast, chopped

6 tbsp. MCT oil (unflavored)

Combine beans, water, stock, half of the onions, and garlic in a large pot and bring to a boil. Reduce heat, cover, and simmer until onions are soft.

Heat 3 tbsp. MCT oil in a skillet. Add remaining chopped onion, chili peppers, and spices. Cook until tender. Add this mixture, plus cooked turkey, to the pot and cook 30 minutes on moderate heat.

Makes 6 servings.
450 calories per serving; 16 grams of fat per serving.

◆ ◆ ◆

Home Fries

3 medium potatoes, sliced
3 tbsp. MCT oil (unflavored)
1/2 tsp. onion powder
1/2 tsp. garlic powder
Dash of red pepper
1/4 cup water

Place all ingredients except water in a large glass bowl and toss until potatoes are evenly coated with oil and spices. Place in a hot nonstick skillet, cover, and cook on medium heat for about 5 minutes.

Pour water in skillet and turn potatoes with spatula. Cover again and cook until potatoes are tender and lightly browned, stirring occasionally.

Makes 3 servings.
266 calories per serving; 14 grams of fat per serving.

◆ ◆ ◆

Fried Squash

2 cups summer squash, cut into strips
1 egg white

Chili powder to taste

Pepper to taste

1½ cups oatmeal, ground fine in the blender

⅓ cup water

4 tbsp. MCT oil

Preheat oven to 425 degrees. Mix all ingredients together except squash strips to form a batter. Dip strips into batter to coat. Spray cookie sheet lightly with vegetable oil spray. Place strips on cookie sheet. Bake 10 to 15 minutes or until browned.

Makes 6 servings.
360 calories per serving; 10.8 grams of fat per serving.

◆ ◆ ◆

Stuffed Mushrooms

¾ pound ground turkey

4 cups medium-sized fresh mushrooms

½ cup shredded wheat, crumbled

1 tsp. Mrs. Dash seasoning

2 tbsp. MCT oil (unflavored)

Parsley to taste

Place MCT oil in a frying pan. Add turkey and brown over medium heat. Add shredded wheat and Mrs. Dash seasoning. Cook for 5 minutes, then remove pan from heat.

Remove stems from mushrooms. Wash mushroom caps thoroughly and place on a cookie sheet that has been sprayed with vegetable spray. Spoon turkey mixture into mushroom caps and bake for 10 minutes, or until mushrooms are brown and tender. Garnish with parsley.

_____

Makes 4 servings.
187 calories per serving; 11 grams of fat per serving.

◆ ◆ ◆

MCT Raspberry Vinaigrette

1 cup MCT oil (unflavored)

³⁄₄ cup raspberry vinegar

1 tbsp. Dijon mustard

1 tbsp. honey

1 tbsp. shallots, minced

Mix ingredients completely in a glass container with a tight-fitting lid. Shake well and serve over salads. 124 calories in each tablespoon.

◆ ◆ ◆

Garlic Lover's MCT Oil Pesto

¹⁄₃ cup chopped fresh basil

¹⁄₄ cup minced garlic

2 tbsp. chopped onion

1 tbsp. MCT oil (unflavored)
Pinch of salt if desired.

Sauté all ingredients in a small nonstick frying pan.
Pesto can be served over rice, pasta, or chicken.

Makes 1 serving.
134 calories per serving; 14 grams of fat per serving.

◆ ◆ ◆

Mexican Bean Dip

1¼ cup cooked pinto beans, washed and drained
1 large tomato, finely chopped
4 tbsp. MCT oil (unflavored)
½ tsp. chili powder
½ tsp. cumin

Purée beans in a food processor or blender, or mash
with a fork. Add rest the ingredients and continue to
blend.

◆ ◆ ◆

Corn Chips

½ cup boiling water
2 tbsp. MCT oil (unflavored)
1 cup cornmeal
¼ tsp. chili powder
Popcorn salt

Preheat oven to 350 degrees. Pour water over MCT oil, cornmeal, and chili powder. Mix well with a fork. Shape dough into small one-inch balls and place far enough apart on a nonstick cookie sheet so that they do not touch when pressed flat. Press balls as flat and as thinly as you can, shaping them into triangles, ovals, or rectangles. Sprinkle lightly with pinches of popcorn salt. Bake about 30 minutes or until edges start to brown. Chips should be thin and crisp. Serve with Mexican Bean Dip.

♦ ♦♦ ♦

Potato Chips

2 medium potatoes, with or without skin

1 tbsp. MCT oil (unflavored)

Pinch of garlic powder

Popcorn salt to taste

Preheat oven to 325 degrees. Slice potatoes very thinly—thin enough so that they are almost transparent. Soak slices in MCT oil and garlic powder for 15 minutes. Place potato slices on a nonstick 14 × 10-inch baking sheet. Do not overlap them. Sprinkle with pinches of popcorn salt. Bake for 30 minutes, or until edges and smaller slices are browned. Remove from cookie sheet and drain on a paper towel.

Variation: Try flavoring your chips with barbecue seasoning powder instead of garlic.

OLIVE OIL RECIPES

From olives and olive oil come some of the most nutri-
tious substances on the planet, namely heart-healthy
monounsaturated fatty acids and antioxidants. Olive oil is
a terrific cooking oil because it can withstand higher cooking temperatures and is slow to oxidize, with little production of disease-causing free radicals.

The following olive oil recipes, rich in not only monounsaturated fats but also in omega-3 fats, are used with
permission from the California Olive Industry, 1903 North
Fine #102, Fresno, California 93727, 559-456-9099,
www.calolive.org.

Salmon with Pine Nut–Rosemary Olive Crust

¾ cup ripe olives

**½ cup pine nuts (filberts or pecans may be substituted
for pine nuts)**

1 tablespoon fresh chopped rosemary

4 (6–8 oz.) portions of salmon or halibut fillets/steaks

To taste, salt and pepper

In a food processor bowl fitted with a blade, pulse
olives until finely chopped; transfer to a shallow bowl.
Pulse pine nuts in a food processor bowl until minced;
transfer to olive bowl. Blend rosemary into pine nut–
olive mixture.

Season salmon with salt and pepper, if desired. Press
½-cup portions of olive mixture onto the surface of
each fish fillet. Bake on spray-coated tray in 450 de-

gree oven for 15 to 20 minutes, or until fish is firm.

Makes 4 servings.
475 calories per serving; 31 grams of fat per serving (16 grams of monounsaturated fat).

♦ ♦ ♦

Shellfish Fettuccine with Ripe Olives and Garlic

¼ cup olive oil

3 pounds Roma tomatoes, diced

½ cup capers

¼ cup anchovies, chopped

2 tbsp. garlic, chopped

1 six-ounce can California Ripe Olives, whole, pitted

3 pounds shrimp, medium, peeled, deveined

2 one-lb. packages fettuccine pasta, cooked, hot

2 tbsp. olive oil

½ cup flat-leaf parsley, fresh, chopped

Heat olive oil in shallow heavy pot. Add tomatoes, capers, anchovies, and garlic. Cook over medium heat until tomatoes release juices and mixture thickens, about 5 to 10 minutes. Add olives and shrimp. Simmer until shrimp is firm, about 4 to 5 minutes. Toss hot pasta with olive oil. Add shrimp mixture to hot pasta and toss well. Portion onto plates or shallow bowls. Sprinkle with chopped parsley.

Makes 8 servings.

430 calories per serving; 18 grams of fat per serving (11 grams of monounsaturated fat).

❖ ❖ ❖

California Black Olive Pesto

1 cup California Ripe Olives (pitted)

⅓ cup chopped fresh basil leaves

⅛ cup pine nuts

½ cup olive oil

¼ cup Parmesan cheese, grated

⅛ teaspoon pepper

Place olives, basil, and nuts in a food processor and pulse, until finely chopped. Slowly add olive oil while still pulsing. Add Parmesan, plus pepper.

Makes 4 servings.
362 calories per serving; 40.65 grams of fat per serving (27.65 grams of monounsaturated fat).

❖ ❖ ❖

White Bean and Ripe Olive Gratin

2 tbsp. olive oil

1 cup celery, thinly sliced

½ cup red onion, thinly sliced

1 tsp. garlic, minced

2 cups each: Roma tomatoes, seeded and diced; and zucchini, ¼-inch sliced

2 cups California Ripe Olives, sliced

¼ cup fresh sage, chopped

2 fifteen-oz. cans white beans, rinsed

1 cup bread crumbs, fresh

1 tsp. garlic

¼ cup parsley, chopped

1 tsp. lemon zest, grated

2 tbsp. olive oil

Preheat oven to 350 degrees. Heat olive oil in heavy pot. Add celery, onions, and garlic. Sauté over medium-high heat for 3 minutes. Add tomatoes and zucchini and simmer for 5 minutes. Remove from heat. Add olives and sage. Purée about ¼ of the beans and add all beans to the tomato mixture. Mix well and adjust seasoning with salt and pepper.

Transfer to a buttered 2-quart shallow baking dish. Combine the last five ingredients in a small bowl. Mix well and sprinkle evenly over casserole. Bake at 350 degrees until bubbly and golden, about 45 minutes. Let rest 5 or 10 minutes prior to serving.

_____

Makes 8 servings.
321 calories per serving; 17 grams of fat per serving (11 grams of monounsaturated fat).

• • •

Mediterranean Baked Zucchini

1 cup California Ripe Olive wedges

2 tbsp. chopped parsley

1 tablespoon chopped scallion greens

1 tbsp. lemon juice

6 Roma tomatoes (sliced)

3 medium zucchini (sliced)

2 tbsp. olive oil

1/2 tsp. salt

1/4 tsp. black pepper

Combine first four ingredients in a small bowl. Layer tomato and zucchini slices in a casserole dish sprayed with nonstick spray. Sprinkle olive oil mixture over the top. Sprinkle with olive oil, salt, and pepper.

Bake in a preheated 350 degree oven until zucchini is tender, about 15 to 20 minutes.

Makes 6 servings.
130 calories per serving; 11 grams of fat per serving (7 grams of monounsaturated fat).

• • •

Olive Caesar Salad

Garlic croutons (recipe follows)

1 large egg

1/4 cup olive oil

1 clove garlic, minced

12 cups rinsed and crisped bite-size pieces romaine lettuce

Pepper

2 tbsp. lemon juice

¾ cup California Ripe Olives, wedged

3 to 4 canned anchovy fillets, chopped

¼ cup grated Parmesan cheese

Prepare garlic croutons; set aside. Immerse egg in boiling water to cover for exactly 1 minute; remove from water and set aside. Beat to blend oil and garlic in a large serving bowl. Add lettuce with a few croutons and pepper; mix gently but thoroughly. Break coddled egg over salad and sprinkle with lemon juice; mix well. Add olives, anchovies, and cheese; mix again. Add remaining croutons; mix gently. Serve immediately.

Garlic croutons: In a 9-inch pan, combine 1 tablespoon olive oil with 1 clove garlic, minced. Add 1 cup ¾-inch cubes day-old French bread and mix to coat. Bake bread cubes in a 325-degree oven until crisp and tinged with brown, 15 to 20 minutes; stir occasionally.

Makes about 14 cups salad; 8 servings.
144 calories per serving; 13 grams of fat per serving (8 grams of monounsaturated fat).

• • •

Couscous Salad with Ripe Olives and Roasted Vegetables

2 cups California Ripe Olives, halved

8 cups couscous, prepared, chilled

2 tsp. thyme, fresh, chopped

1 tsp. rosemary, fresh, chopped

½ cup red wine vinaigrette dressing

¼ cup capers

2 large zucchini, ½-inch lengthwise, sliced

3 large leeks, white only, lengthwise split

2 red bell peppers, seeded, quartered

10 garlic cloves, peeled

¼ cup olive oil

Preheat oven to 400 degrees F. Combine first six ingredients in large bowl. Cover and set aside. Arrange zucchini, leeks, bell pepper, and garlic on roasting pan. Brush with olive oil and sprinkle as desired with salt and pepper. Roast in preheated oven until tender, about 35 to 40 minutes. Cool vegetables and cut into ½-inch dices; chop garlic. Add vegetables to reserved couscous mixture. Toss gently but well. Chill completely. Remove from refrigerator 30 minutes before serving.

Makes 8 servings.
375 calories per serving; 16.5 grams of fat per serving (10.5 grams of monounsaturated fat).

❖ ❖ ❖

ADDITIONAL GOOD FAT RECIPES

The following recipes are some of my personal favorites for using healthy ingredients such as flaxseeds, flaxseed oil, sesame seeds, sesame oil, and canola oil.

Natural Muffins

1 cup oatmeal flour

1 cup cornmeal

1 tbsp. baking powder

1/2 tsp. salt

3 egg whites

2 tbsp. honey

3 tbsp. canola oil

1 cup skim milk

1/2 cup flaxseeds

Mix dry ingredients (flour, cornmeal, baking power, and salt) together. In a separate bowl, blend the remaining ingredients and pour into the dry mixture. Blend thoroughly. Pour batter into muffin tins that have been sprayed with vegetable spray or into cupcake papers. Bake at 400 degrees for 20 to 25 minutes or until brown.

_____

Makes 1 dozen muffins, which can be served at breakfast, for snacks, or at other meals.
120 calories per muffin; 4 grams of fat per muffin.

• • •

Low-Fat Flaxseed Apricot Bread

1½ cups oatmeal flour

1 tbsp. baking powder

1 tsp. baking soda

½ tsp. salt

1 tsp. cinnamon

1½ cups wheat bran

1 package dried apricots, cut into bits

½ cup unsweetened applesauce

1 cup boiling water

½ cup reduced-calorie maple syrup (fructose sweetened)

2 egg whites

½ cup flaxseeds

1 tsp. vanilla

Stir together oatmeal flour, baking powder, baking soda, salt, and cinnamon. In a separate bowl, combine bran, apricots, applesauce, and water. Stir well. In another bowl, blend egg whites, syrup, and vanilla. Add contents of both bowls to the dry mixture and blend well. Pour batter into a loaf pan that has been coated with vegetable spray. Bake for 1 hour in a 375-degree oven. Remove from oven and refrigerate. Slice bread when cool.

_____

Makes 12 slices.
104 calories per slice; 1.5 grams of fat.

◆ ◆ ◆

Quick Gourmet Flaxseed Oil Dressing

¼ cup white balsamic vinegar

3 tablespoons water

1 package (0.75 oz.) Good Seasonings Garlic & Herb salad dressing mix

½ cup flaxseed oil

Place vinegar and water in a container with a tight-fitting lid. Add salad dressing mix and shake vigorously until well blended. Add oil and shake again until well blended. Can be refrigerated for up to four weeks.

---

70 calories per tablespoon; 7.5 grams of fat per tablespoon.

• • •

Sesame Cheese Hors d'Oeuvres

1 eight-oz. package fat-free cream cheese

Soy sauce

Sesame seeds

With a toothpick, poke holes in the cream cheese. Slowly pour soy sauce over the cream cheese so that the soy sauce flows into the holes. Roll the cream cheese in sesame seeds so that it is completely coated with seeds. Refrigerate. Serve with wheat crackers.

• • •

Mediterranean Salad

¹/₂ cup garbanzo beans

2 oz. feta cheese

¹/₂ onion, chopped

¹/₂ red pepper, chopped

Lettuce

Quick Gourmet Flaxseed Oil Dressing

Arrange beans, cheese, onion, and red pepper on a bed of lettuce. Drizzle with 1 tbsp. of salad dressing.

Makes 1 serving.
543 calories per serving; 23 grams of fat per serving.

◆ ◆ ◆

Chicken Broccoli Orientale

2 tbsp. cornstarch

6 tbsp. soy sauce

1 package skinless chicken breasts (about 4), cut in cubes

¹/₄ cup white wine

4 tsp. brown sugar

2 tsp. vinegar

2 tbsp. sesame oil

2 tsp. crushed red pepper

1 tbsp. chopped garlic

2 medium onions, cut into chunks

1 lb. bag frozen broccoli cuts

Blend cornstarch and 4 tbsp. soy sauce in a bowl. Add chicken and stir to coat. Mix the rest of the soy sauce with wine, brown sugar, and vinegar. Set aside. Heat oil in wok at 300 degrees and add red pepper and garlic. Cook for 1 minute. Add chicken. Stir-fry until chicken is cooked. Add onion and broccoli. Cover wok and cook mixture until broccoli is tender—about 5 minutes, stirring occasionally. Remove cover and add wine mixture. Cook until sauce becomes thickened—3 to 4 minutes. Serve over hot rice.

Makes 4 servings.
276 calories; 11 grams of fat per serving.

◆ ◆ ◆

A COOKING OIL PRIMER

Today, more than any other time in culinary history, there is a huge array of oils that can be used in cooking. To enhance and maximize flavor, it helps to know which oils are best for which types of recipes. Box 15 provides an at-a-glance review of various cooking oils, their characteristics and uses.

Low-Fat Cooking

Perhaps for medical reasons, you have been told to reduce the amount of fat in your diet. Here are some tips for cutting fat in recipes, without sacrificing flavor:

• Trim the fat from any meat before cooking. The skin from poultry can be removed after cooking.

Table 15

USING COOKING OILS

Oil	Characteristics	Uses
Almond oil	Tastes slightly al-mond.	Making pastry.
Avocado oil	Smooth, rich taste.	Salad dressing, bread dipping, stir-frying.
Canola oil	Lowest of all oils in saturated fat; mild-tasting.	Salads, baking, deep-fat frying, stir-frying.
Corn oil	All-purpose oil.	Salad dressings, mayonnaise, deep-frying.
Flaxseed oil	Pungent flavor.	Salad dressings.
Hazelnut oil	Nutty flavor.	Salad dressings.
Olive oil	Comes in several forms.	Salad dressings, mayonnaise, bread dipping, cooking (but not baking).
Peanut oil	Mild flavor.	Stir-frying, deep-frying.
Rice oil	Sweet taste.	Salad dressings, cooking.

- Brown meats by broiling, grilling, or cooking in non-stick pans with little or no oil.

- Cook meat, poultry, and fish so that fat drains off.

- Use nonstick vegetable sprays because they reduce the amount of oil or shortening required for cooking.

- Marinate meat, fish, and poultry in low-fat or nonfat salad dressings for added flavor.

- Substitute low-fat milk for whole milk in recipes.

Table 15 continued

USING COOKING OILS

Oil	Characteristics	Uses
Safflower oil	Mild taste.	Salad dressings, stir-frying, all-purpose cooking.
Sesame oil	Comes in light (made from un-toasted seeds) and dark (made from toasted seeds); nutty flavor.	Light version is good for frying, grilling, and in marinades. Dark version is good for flavoring foods, not for cooking.
Soybean oil	Light and mild-tasting.	Salad dressings, sautéing, deep-frying.
Sunflower oil	Bland flavor.	Salad dressings, all-purpose cooking.
Walnut oil	Light and mild-tasting; tastes like walnuts; goes rancid quickly.	Salad dressings.
Wheat germ oil	Nutty flavor, very high in vitamin E.	Salad dressings.

- Shun nondairy creamers and toppings, which are high in saturated tropical oils.

- Sauté vegetables in broth, bouillon, or wine, rather than in butter, margarine, or oil.

- Substitute low-fat yogurt, buttermilk, or low-fat cottage cheese for sour cream in recipes.

- Substitute the fat or oil with an equal amount of applesauce or fruit pureé in baked products. Both are wonderful replacements for the fat in baked products such as quick breads.

- For sauces and dressings, use low-calorie bases such as vinegar, mustard, tomato juice, and fat-free bouillon, instead of high-calorie ones like creams, fats, oils, and mayonnaise.

- You can reduce the amount of fat or oil in most recipes by about a third without affecting the recipe.

- When making soups, stews, sauces, and broths, you can remove 100 calories of fat per tablespoon by chilling the liquid after cooking and skimming off the congealed fat.

- Use low-fat cheeses in place of regular cheeses in recipes.

- Use egg whites or egg substitutes to replace whole eggs in recipes.

- 3 tablespoons of cocoa powder, plus 1 tablespoon of vegetable oil, can replace 1 ounce of baking chocolate in recipes.

Glossary

ALKYLGLYCEROLS. A group of lipids similar in structure to triglycerides that are found in other fatty fish, as well as in human bone marrow and breast milk. Alkylglycerols have been scientifically studied since the 1930s for their ability to reduce radiation damage, suppress tumor growth, build blood, and accelerate wound healing.

ALPHA-LINOLENIC FATTY ACID (ALA). An omega-3 fatty acid found mostly in vegetables, nuts, seeds, and oils produced from those sources.

ANTIOXIDANT. A special class of nutrients that fight *free radicals,* unstable molecules that damage otherwise healthy cells.

ARACHIDONIC ACID (AA). A fatty acid found mostly in animal foods, but also synthesized from the omega-6 fat, linoleic acid, in a process involving enzymes. Arachidonic acid can be converted to bad prostaglandins and leukotrienes in the body.

ATHEROSCLEROSIS. Narrowing and thickening of the arteries caused by deposits of cholesterol, fats, and other substances.

BLACK CURRANT SEED OIL. A rich source of alpha-linolenic acid and gamma-linolenic acid (GLA).

BORAGE OIL. A highly concentrated source of gamma-linolenic acid (GLA).

CALORIES. Units that represent the amount of energy provided by food.

CANOLA OIL. A healthy monounsaturated fat extracted from the seeds of the rapeseed plant.

CHOLESTEROL. A fatty substance found in some foods and manufactured by the body for many vital functions. Excess cholesterol and saturated fat can increase blood levels of cholesterol and can collect inside artery walls. This process contributes to heart disease.

CONJUGATED LINOLEIC ACID (CLA). A naturally occurring fatty acid present in dairy products (most notably milk fat) as well as in meat, sunflower oil, and safflower oil. It is formed when the bacteria in a cow's gut breaks down the essential fatty acid, linoleic acid, in the food the animal eats. Marketed as a natural fat-loss supplement.

DIHOMO-GAMMA LINOLENIC ACID (DGLA). A fatty acid that is synthesized from gamma-linolenic acid (GLA) in an enzyme-controlled process. DGLA is converted to good prostaglandins in the body, but can also be converted to arachidonic acid.

DOCOSAHEXAENOIC ACID (DHA). An important fatty acid constituent of the brain and retina. Fish is a rich source of DHA.

EICOSANOIDS. Hormonelike substances that are produced in the body from fats. They include prostaglandins and leukotrienes.

EICOSAPENTAENOIC ACID (EPA). A very potent fatty acid that prevents platelets in the blood from abnormal clotting, and also helps reduce inflammation. Alpha-linolenic acid is converted to EPA in the body.

ESSENTIAL FATTY ACIDS (EFAS). Vitaminlike substances that have a protective effect on the body. They are called essential because the body cannot manufacture them. They must be obtained from food.

EVENING PRIMROSE OIL. A supplement made from the seeds of the evening primrose plant that is valued for its GLA content.

FAT REPLACERS. Food additives concocted from carbohydrates, protein, and other fats to replace the fat in foods.

FATS. A food group that provides energy and is the most concentrated source of calories in the diet.

FATTY ACID CHAIN. Carbon atoms with hydrogen atoms attached and with an acid group at one end.

FATTY ACIDS. A building block of either dietary fat or body fat.

FLAX. A plant whose seeds yield a high amount of alpha-linolenic acid.

FREE RADICALS. Cellular aberrations, formed when molecules somehow come up with an odd number of electrons. These cells destroy healthy cells by robbing them of oxygen, and this robbery weakens the immune system.

GAMMA-LINOLENIC ACID (GLA). A fatty acid made from linoleic acid in the body. GLA has a number of benefits, including the ability to fight inflammation.

HDL (HIGH DENSITY LIPOPROTEIN). A type of cholesterol in the blood that protects against the buildup of plaque in the arteries.

HEMPSEED OIL. A nutritional oil made from the seeds of the hemp plant. It is rich in omega-6 fats.

HYDROGENATED FATS. Polyunsaturated omega-6 fatty acids that have been synthetically altered in a process called hydrogenation in which hydrogen is forced into the oil.

HYDROXYTYROSOL. A powerful antioxidant in olives and olive oil that is technically classified as a polyphenol.

LECITHIN. A phospholipid involved in the proper metabolism of cholesterol.

LEUKOTRIENES. Substances in the body that are involved in inflammation. They are produced from fatty acids.

LIGNANS. Plant chemicals that act as antioxidants.

LINOLEIC ACID. An omega-6 fatty acid found in vegetable oils, margarine, and processed foods.

LIPIDS. A family of chemical compounds that generally do not dissolve in water. Examples are fats and oils.

LIPID TRIAD. A risk factor for heart disease characterized by the presence of elevated triglycerides (dietary fats not fully broken down by the liver that circulate in the blood), too-low HDL cholesterol, and high LDL cholesterol—in particular, a type of LDL cholesterol characterized by its small particle size.

LIPOPROTEINS. Protein blankets that carry fats to their destinations in the body.

MCT OIL (MEDIUM-CHAIN TRIGLYCERIDE OIL). A dietary fat metabolized in such a way that very little is stored as body fat.

MICELLE. A tiny droplet made of lipids and emulsifiers from bile. They package cholesterol for transport in the body.

MONOUNSATURATED FAT. Fatty acids that lack two hydrogen atoms. Found in such foods as olives, olive oil, avocados, cashew nuts, and cold-water fish such as salmon, mackerel, halibut, and swordfish.

OLEIC ACID. A monounsaturated fat found most notably in olive oil.

OLEUROPEIN. The most abundant polyphenol, an antioxidantlike substance, found in olives and olive oil.

OLIVE OIL. A healthy monounsaturated fat pressed from olives.

OMEGA-3 FATTY ACIDS. Essential fats found in fish and plants that appear to prevent blood clots and the buildup of plaque on arterial walls. Omega-3 fatty acids also play a role in strengthening the immune system.

OMEGA-6 FATTY ACIDS. Essential fats that are generally necessary for normal growth, hair and skin health, regulation of metabolism, and reproduction.

OXIDATION. A chemical process in which oxygen combines with another substance, which is changed to another form.

PERILLA OIL. A supplement oil containing high amounts of alpha-linolenic acid.

PHOSPHOLIPIDS. Fatlike substances that contain a molecule of phosphorus, which makes them soluble in water. This characteristic helps fats travel in and out of the lipid-rich membranes of cells.

PLANT STEROLS. Naturally occurring substances present in small quantities in many fruits, vegetables, legumes, nuts, seeds, grains, and other plant sources. Used in cholesterol-lowering margarines.

PLATELETS. Tiny clotting factors in blood.

POLYPHENOLS. Disease-fighting substances that play roles in cardiovascular health and cancer protection.

POLYUNSATURATED FAT. A fatty acid that lacks four or more hydrogen atoms. Found in fish and in most vegetable oils.

PROSTACYCLIN. Synthesized mostly from EPA, prostacyclin orders platelets to not stick together and move along.

PROSTAGLANDINS. Hormonelike compounds made from fatty acids that regulate nearly every system in the body.

SATURATED FAT. A fatty acid that is solid at room temperature.

SATURATION. The number of hydrogens in a fatty acid chain.

SESAME OIL. A cooking oil extracted from sesame seeds. It contains a powerful antioxidant called sesaminol.

SQUALENE. A vitaminlike chemical found in olives, olive oil, and shark liver oil.

STEARIC ACID. A saturated fat that does not cause heart problems.

STEARIDONIC ACID. A by-product of alpha-linolenic acid that may be responsible for many of the health benefits associated with black currant seed oil.

THROMBOXANE. A prostaglandin mainly synthesized from arachidonic acid that tells platelets—tiny clotting factors in your blood—to clump together.

TRANS-FATTY ACIDS. By-products of hydrogenation that are responsible for causing serious diseases.

TRIGLYCERIDES. Fats that circulate in the blood until they are deposited in fat cells. Triglycerides make up about 95 percent of dietary fat and 90 percent of body fat.

TROPICAL OILS. A group of vegetable fats that are saturated. They include coconut oil, palm and palm kernel oils, and the cocoa butter in chocolate.

TYROSOL. A major polyphenol in olives and olive oil. It functions as an antioxidant to help prevent the oxidation of LDL cholesterol and keep free radicals from attacking cell membranes.

UNSATURATED FAT. Fats that are liquid at room temperature.

VERY-LOW-DENSITY LIPOPROTEINS. A harmful type of cholesterol.

WHEAT GERM OIL. Extracted from wheat germ and sold as a nutritional supplement, wheat germ oil contains a number of healthful substances, including octacosanol, an alcohol derivative that may be heart-healthy; vitamin E, an important antioxidant; and several minerals.

References

A portion of the information in this book comes from medical research reports in both popular and scientific publications, professional textbooks and booklets, promotional literature from supplement companies, case studies, Internet sources, and computer searches of medical databases of research abstracts.

Chapter 1. The Fats of Life

Carper, J. 1995. *Stop aging now!* New York: Harper-Perennial.

Editor. 2001. Frequently asked questions. Online: www.fatsforhealth.com.

Herbert, V. (ed.). 1995. *Total nutrition: The only guide you'll ever need*. New York: St. Martin's Press.

Kettler, D. B. 2001. Can manipulation of the ratios of essential fatty acids slow the rapid rate of postmenopausal bone loss? *Alternative Medicine Review* 6: 61–77.

Lawton, C. L., et al. 2000. The degree of saturation of fatty acids influences post-ingestive satiety. *British Journal of Nutrition* 83: 473–482.

Murray, M. T. 1996. *Encyclopedia of nutritional supplements*. Rocklin, California: Prima Publishing.

Sizer, F., and E. Whitney. 1997. *Nutrition concepts and controversies*. 7th ed. Belmont, California: West/Wadsworth.

Chapter 2. When Fat Can Be Fatal

Applegate, L. 1994. Fat transformed. *Runner's World,* February, pp. 26–27.

Carper, J. 1995. *Stop aging now!* New York: Harper-Perennial.

Chong, Y. H., et al. 1991. Effects of palm oil on cardiovascular risk. *The Medical Journal of Malaysia* 46: 41–50.

Collins, S. 2001. Your health: Chocolate is good for you. *Sunday Mirror,* April 15, pp. 44–45.

Connor, W. E. 1999. Harbingers of coronary heart disease: dietary saturated fatty acids and cholesterol. Is chocolate benign because of its stearic acid content? *American Journal of Clinical Nutrition* 70: 951–952.

De La Taille, A., et al. 2001. Cancer of the prostate: influence of nutritional factors. General nutritional factors. *Presse Medicale* 30: 554–556.

Ebong, P. E., et al. 1999. Influence of palm oil (Elaesis guineensis) on health. *Plant Foods for Human Nutrition* 53: 209–222.

Editor. 1996. The good news about "bad" foods. *Good Housekeeping*, September, pp. 93–94.

Editor. 1992. Relax, Mrs. Sprat high-fat, low-fiber diets may not cause breast cancer after all. *Time,* November 2, p. 23.

Editor. 1998. Researchers sweet on health benefits of chocolate (stearic acid). Medical *Post,* September 22, p. 59.

Elson, C. E. 1992. Tropical oils: nutritional and scientific issues. *Critical Reviews in Food and Science Nutrition* 31: 79–102.

Eritson, J. 2000. Safety considerations of polyunsaturated fatty acids. *American Journal of Clinical Nutrition* 71: 197–201.

Fallon, S., et al. 1996. Diet and heart disease: not what you think. *Consumers' Research Magazine,* July, pp. 15–19.

Fallon, S. 1996. Why butter is good for you. *Consumers' Research Magazine*, March, pp. 10–15.

Herbert, V. (ed.). 1995. *Total nutrition: The only guide you'll ever need.* New York: St. Martin's Press.

Hooper, J. 1998. What you still don't know about cholesterol. *Esquire,* March, pp. 136–138.

Lichtenstein, A. H., et al. Dietary fat consumption and health. *Nutrition Reviews* 56: S3–S28.

Murray, M. T. 1996. *Encyclopedia of nutritional supplements.* Rocklin, California: Prima Publishing.

Nash, J. M. 1994. Is a low-fat diet risky? *Time,* September 5, p. 62.

Sadler, C. 1998. The fat came back. *Chatelaine,* April, pp. 163–164.

Sizer, F., and E. Whitney. 1997. *Nutrition concepts and controversies.* 7th ed. Belmont, California: West/Wadsworth.

Stampfer, M. J., et al. 2000. Primary prevention of coronary heart disease in women through diet and lifestyle. *New England Journal of Medicine* 343: 16–22.

Wells, A. S., et al. 1998. Alterations in mood after changing to a low-fat diet. *British Journal of Nutrition* 79: 23–30.

Chapter 3. Fishing for Good Health

Appel, A. 1999. A fish tale. *Natural Health,* April. Online: www.findarticles.com.

Appel, L. J., et al. 1993. Does supplementation of diet with fish oil reduce blood pressure? A meta-analysis of controlled clinical trials. *Archives of Internal Medicine* 153: 1429–1438.

Applegate, L. 1999. Make room for fish. *Runner's World*, October, pp. 26–28.

Belluzzi, A., et al. 2000. Polyunsaturated fatty acids and inflammatory bowel disease. *American Journal of Clinical Nutrition* 71: 339S–342S.

Brewer, S. 2001. Family health. *Daily Record,* February 28, p. 6.

Bucci, L. 1993. Nutrients as ergogenic aids for sports and exercise. Boca Raton, Florida: CRC Press.

Carper, J. 1995. *Stop aging now*! New York: Harper-Perennial.

Connor, W. E., et al. 1993. N-3 fatty acids from fish oil. *Annals of the New York Academy of Sciences* 683: 16–34.

Durham, J. 1999. The skinny on fat. *Saturday Evening Post,* May.

Editor. 1997. Schizophrenia symptoms eased with fish oil. *Medical Post,* September 9, p. 61.

Freeman, M. P. 2000. Omega-3 fatty acids in psychiatry: a review. *Annals of Clinical Psychiatry* 12: 159–165.

Goodman, J. 2001. *The omega solution*. Rocklin, California: Prima Publishing.

Gorman, C., et al. 2000. They're full of a special fat called omega-3 that may actually be good for you. *Time*, October 30, p. 76.

Halpern, G. M. 2000. Anti-inflammatory effects of a stabilized lipid extract of Perna canaliculus (Lyprinol). *Allergie et Immunologie* 32: 272–278.

Herbert, V. (ed.). 1995. *Total nutrition: The only guide you'll ever need*. New York: St. Martin's Press.

Jobrin, J. 1996. Tackle arthritis with a knife and fork. *Prevention*, November, pp. 83–91.

Joy, C. B., et al. 2000. Polyunsaturated fatty fish (fish or evening primrose oil) for schizophrenia. Cochrane Database System Review.

Kremer, J. M., et al. 1995. Effects of high-dose fish oil on rheumatoid arthritis after stopping nonsteroidal antiinflammatory drugs. Clinical and immune correlates. *Arthritis and Rheumatism* 38: 1107–1114.

Leaf, A. 1992. The role of omega-3 fatty acids in the prevention and rehabilitation of coronary artery disease. *Annals of the Academy of Medicine* 21: 132–136.

McCord, H. 1999. Nutrition news: this oil's a lifesaver. *Prevention*, October, p. 56.

McCord, H. 1997. The fat you need. *Prevention,* January, pp. 100–108.

Nettleton, J. A. 1991. Omega-3 fatty acids: comparison of plant and seafood sources. *Journal of the American Dietetic Association* 91: 331–337.

Pugliese, P. T., et al. 1998. Some biological actions of alkylglycerols from shark liver oil. *Journal of Alternative and Complementary Medicine* 4: 87–99.

SerVaas, C., et al. 1999. Fats for mental health. *Saturday Evening Post,* March.

Simopoulos, A. P. 1999. Evolutionary aspects of omega-3 fatty acids in the food supply. *Prostaglandins, Leukotrienes, and Essential Fatty Acids* 60: 421–429.

Sinclair, A. J., et al. 2000. Marine lipids: overview "new insights and lipid composition of Lyprinol." *Allergie et Immunologie* 32: 261–271.

Webb, D. 1999. Healthy diet: the smart fat makeover. *Prevention,* April, pp. 134–141.

Webb, D. 2000. Can fish oil chase away both heart attacks and blues? *Prevention,* March, pp. 69–70.

Yetiv, J. Z. 1988. Clinical applications of fish oil. *Journal of the American Medical Association* 260: 665–670.

Chapter 4. DHA: The Brain-Building Fat

Brody, J. 2001. Science sees new diet role in eye care. *Minneapolis Star Tribune,* March 21, p. 04E.

Cooper, R. 1998. *DHA: the essential omega-3 fatty acid.* Pleasant Grove, Utah.

Dickstein, L. 1999. DHA: the good fat. *Psychology Today,* April, p. 50.

Editor. 1997. Alzheimer's, depression, attention-deficit/hyperactivity disorder linked to low levels of DHA, a key brain fat. April 9. Online: www.royal-health.com.

Editor. 2001. DHA: the mind mender. *Psychology Today,* March, p. 48.

Editor. 1997. Lack of breast milk may be risk factor in schizophrenia. May 15. Online: www.royal-health.com.

Editor. 1995. Two studies report Martek's DHA—Neuromins™—improves HDL:LDL cholesterol ration and lowers triglycerides. July 11. Online: www.royal-health.com.

Gamoh, S., et al. 1999. Chronic administration of docosahexaenoic acid improves reference memory–related learning ability in young rats. *Neuroscience* 93: 237–241.

Horrocks, L. A., et al. 1999. Health benefits of docosahexaenoic acid (DHA). *Pharmacological Research* 40: 211–225.

Mori, T. A., et al. 1999. Docosahexaenoic acid but not eicosapentaenoic acid lowers ambulatory blood pressure and heart rate in humans. *Hypertension* 34: 253–260.

Murray, M. T. 1999. Must-have nutrients for mothers-to-be. *Better Nutrition,* August. Online: www.findarticles.com.

Shimura, T., et al. 1997. Docosahexaenoic acid (DHA) improved glucose and lipid metabolism in KK-Ay mice with genetic non-insulin-dependent diabetes mellitus (NIDDM). *Biological & Pharmaceutical Bulletin* 20: 507–510.

Waltman, A. B., et al. 2000. Guide to natural health: alternative medicine goes mainstream. *Psychology Today,* April, pp. 37–40, 42.

Chapter 5. Nature's Disease Fighters

Allman, M. A., et al. 1995. Supplementation with flaxseed oil versus sunflower seed oil in healthy young men consuming a low fat diet: effects on platelet composition and function. *European Journal of Clinical Nutrition* 49: 169–178.

American Lung Association. 2001. Acute respiratory distress syndrome (ARDS). Online: www.lungusa.org.

Annuseek, G. 2001. Flaxseed. *Gale Encyclopedia of Alternative Medicine.* Online: www.findarticles.com.

Blumenthal, M. 1998. *The complete German Commission E monographs: therapeutic guide to herbal medicines.* American Botanical Council: Austin, Texas.

Craig, W. J. 1999. Health-promoting properties of common herbs. *American Journal of Clinical Nutrition* 70: 491S–499S.

Cunnane, S. C., et al. 1993. High alpha-linolenic acid flaxseed (linum usitatissimum): some nutritional properties in humans. *British Journal of Nutrition* 69: 443–453.

Editor. 1999. Foods that fight breast cancer. *Saturday Evening Post,* January.

Engler, M. M., et al. 1998. Dietary borage oil alters plasma, hepatic and vascular tissue fatty acid composition in spontaneously hypertensive rats. *Prostaglandins, Leukotrienes, and Essential Fatty Acids* 59: 11–15.

Engler, M. M., et al. Dietary gamma-linolenic acid lowers blood pressure and alters aortic reactivity and cholesterol metabolism in hypertension. *Journal of Hypertension* 10: 1197–1204.

Ezaki, O., et al. 1999. Long-term effects of dietary alpha-linolenic acid from perilla oil on serum fatty acids composition and on the risk factors of coronary heart disease in Japanese elderly subjects. *Journal of Nutritional Science and Vitaminology* 45: 759–772.

Flax Council of Canada. 2001. *Flaxseed.* Winnipeg, Canada: Flax Council of Canada.

Grant, S. 1996. The beauty of borage. December 5, *The Evening Post*, p. 23.

Hartman, I. S. 1995. Alpha-linolenic acid: a prevention in secondary coronary events? *Nutrition Reviews* 53: 194–197.

Jacob, J., et al. 2000. Designer and specialty eggs. The Institute of Food and Agricultural Sciences, University of Florida.

James, M. J., et al. 2000. Dietary polyunsaturated fatty acids and inflammatory mediator production. *American Journal of Clinical Nutrition* 71: 343S–348S.

Jenab, M., et al. 1996. The influence of flaxseed and lignans on colon carcinogenesis and beta-glucuronidase activity. *Carcinogenesis* 17: 1343–1348.

Leventhal, L. J., et al. Treatment of rheumatoid arthritis with gammalinolenic acid. *Annals of Internal Medicine* 119: 867–873.

Masataka, O., et al. 1997. Perilla oil prevents the excessive growth of visceral adipose tissue in rats by downregulating adipocyte differentiation. *Journal of Nutrition* 127: 1752–1757.

Medical Economics Company. 2001. *The PDR for Herbal Medicines*. Montvale, New Jersey: Medical Economics Company. Online: www.pdr.net.

Miller, L. G. 1998. Herbal medicinals: selected clinical considerations focusing on known or potential drug-herb interactions. *Archives of Internal Medicine* 158: 2200–2211.

Mills, D. E., et al. 1989. Dietary fatty acid supplementation alters stress reactivity and performance in man. *Journal of Human Hypertension* 3: 111–116.

Murray, M. T. 1996. *Encyclopedia of nutritional supplements*. Rocklin, California: Prima Publishing.

Narisawa, T., et al. 1994. Colon cancer prevention with a small amount of dietary perilla oil high in alpha-linolenic acid in an animal model. *Cancer* 73: 2069–2075.

Okamoto, M., et al. 2000. Effects of dietary supplementation with n-3 fatty acids compared with n-6 fatty acids on bronchial asthma. *Internal Medicine* 39: 107–111.

Prasad, K. 1997. Dietary flax seed in prevention of hypercholesterolemic atherosclerosis. *Atherosclerosis* 132: 69–76.

Prasad, K. 2000. Oxidative stress as a mechanism of diabetes in diabetic BB prone rats: effect of secoisolariciresinol diglucoside (SDG). *Molecular and Cellular Biochemistry* 209: 89–96.

Prasad, K. 1999. Reduction of serum cholesterol and hypercholesterolemic atherosclerosis in rabbits by secoisolariciresinol diglucoside isolated from flaxseed. *Circulation* 99: 1355–1362.

Shahidi, F. 2000. Antioxidant factors in plant foods and selected oilseeds. *Biofactors* 13: 179–185.

Sung, M. K., et al. 1998. Mammalian lignans inhibit the growth of estrogen-independent human colon tumor cells. *Anticancer Research* 18: 1405–1408.

Swift, D. 1999. Natural oil improves odds of ARDS recovery. *Medical Post,* November 17.

Thompson, L. U., et al. 1996. Flaxseed and its lignan and oil components reduce mammary tumor growth at a late stage of *Carcinogenesis* 17: 1373–1376.

Udall, K. G. 1997. *Flaxseed oil.* Pleasant Grove, Utah: Woodland Publishing.

Yan, L., et al. 1998. Dietary flaxseed supplementation and experimental metastasis of melanoma cells in mice. *Cancer Letter* 124: 181–186.

Chapter 6. Omega-6 Healers

Ahn, Y. O. 1997. Diet and stomach cancer in Korea. *International Journal of Cancer* 10: S7–S9.

Blumenthal, M. 1998. *The complete German Commission E monographs: therapeutic guide to herbal medicines.* American Botanical Council: Austin, Texas.

Campbell, E. M., et al. 1997. Premenstrual symptoms in general practice patients. Prevalence and treatment. *Journal of Reproductive Medicine* 42: 637–646.

Cheung, K. L. 1999. Management of cyclical mastalgia in oriental women. *The Australian New Zealand Journal of Surgery* 69: 492–494.

Craig, W. J. 1999. Health-promoting properties of common herbs. *American Journal of Clinical Nutrition* 70: 491S–499S.

Darlington, L. G., et al. 2001. Antioxidants and fatty acids in the amelioration of rheumatoid arthritis and related disorders. *British Journal of Nutrition* 85: 251–269.

Editor. 2001. Consumer guide to wheat germ oil. Online: www.mothernature.com.

Editor. 1998. Hemp without the high. *Soap Perfumery & Cosmetics* 71: 34.

Editor. 1996. How to relieve vaginal dryness. *Meno Times*, June, p. 4.

Gateley, C. A., et al. 1992. Drug treatments for mastalgia: 17 years experience in the Cardiff Mastalgia Clinic. *Journal of the Royal Society of Medicine* 85: 12–15.

Gateley, C. A., et al. 1991. Management of the painful and modular breast. *British Medical Bulletin* 47: 284–294.

Hardy, M. L. 2000. Herbs of special interest to women. *Journal of the American Pharmaceutical Association* 40: 234–242.

Hilz, M. J., et al. 2000. Diabetic somatic polyneuropathy. *Fortschritte der Neurologie-Psychiatrie* 68: 278–288.

Jill, J. F., et al. 2000. Evening primrose oil and borage oil in rheumatologic conditions. *American Journal of Clinical Nutrition* 71: 352S–356S.

Kagi, M. K., et al. 1993. Falafel burger anaphylaxis due to sesame seed allergy. *Annals of Allergy* 71: 127–129.

Kang, M. H., et al. 2000. Mode of action of sesame lignans in protecting low-density lipoprotein against oxidative damage in vitro. *Life Sciences* 66: 161–171.

Kerscher, M. J., et al. 1992. Treatment of atopic eczema with evening primrose oil: rationale and clinical results. *The Clinical Investigator* 70: 167–171.

Miller, L. G. 1998. Herbal medicinals: selected clinical considerations focusing on known or potential drug-herb interactions. *Archives of Internal Medicine* 158: 2200–2211.

Murray, M. T. 1996. *Encyclopedia of nutritional supplements*. Rocklin, California: Prima Publishing.

Pritchard, G. A., et al. 1989. Lipids in breast carcinogenesis. *British Journal of Surgery* 76: 1069–1073.

Ramesh, G., et al. 1992. Effect of essential fatty acids on tumor cells. *Nutrition* 8: 343–347.

Salerno, J. W., et al. 1991. The use of sesame seed oil and other vegetable oils in the inhibition of human colon cancer growth in vitro. *Anticancer Research* 11: 209–215.

Smith, D. E., et al. 1992. Selective growth inhibition of a human malignant melanoma cell line by sesame in vitro. *Prostaglandins, Leukotrienes, and Essential Fatty Acids* 46: 145–150.

Struempler, R. E. 1997. A positive cannabinoids workplace drug test following the ingestion of commercially available hemp seed oil. *Journal of Analytical Toxicology* 21: 283–285.

Wagner, W., et al. 1997. Prophylactic treatment of migraine with gamma-linolenic and alpha-linolenic acids. *Cephalalgia* 17: 127–130.

Wu, D., et al. 1999. Effect of dietary supplementation with black currant seed oil on the immune response of healthy elderly subjects. *American Journal of Clinical Nutrition* 70: 536–543.

Chapter 7. Olive Oil: The Master Monounsaturated Fat

Ballmer, P. E. 2000. The Mediterranean diet—healthy but still delicious. *Therapeutische Umschau* 57: 167–172.

Bisignano, G., et al. 1999. On the in-vitro antimicrobial activity of oleuropein and hydroxytyrosol. *The Journal of Pharmacy and Pharmacology* 51: 971–974.

California Olive Industry. 2001. Information packet. Fresno, California: California Olive Industry.

California Olive Oil Council. 2000. Health news. Online: www.cooc.com.

Chan, P., et al. 1996. Effectiveness and safety of low-dose pravastatin and squalene, alone and in combination, in elderly patients with hypercholesterolemia. *Journal of Clinical Pharmacology* 36: 422–427.

Covas, M. I., et al. Virgin olive oil phenolic compounds: binding to human low density lipoprotein (LDL) and effect on LDL oxidation. *International Journal of Clinical Pharmacology Research* 20: 49–54.

Dupont, J., et al. 1989. Food safety and health effects on canola oil. *Journal of the American College of Nutrition* 8: 360–375.

Ferrara, L. A., et al. 2000. Olive oil and reduced need for hypertensive medications. *Archives of Internal Medicine* 160: 837–842.

Giovannini, C., et al. 1999. Tyrosol, the major olive oil biophenol, protects against oxidized-LDL-induced injury in caco-2 cells. *Journal of Nutrition* 129: 1269–1277.

Haban, P., et al. 2000. Oleic acid serum phospholipid content is linked with the serum total- and LDL-cholesterol in elderly subjects. *Medical Science Monitor* 6: 1093–1097.

Hammock, D., et al. 2001. Canola oil. May 30. Online: www.goodhousekeeping.women.com.

Horowitz, J. 1990. Food: a card game? No, cooking oil canola is the latest love of the cholesterol-free set. *Time,* November 12, p. 107.

Hunter, B. T. 1999. Modified vegetable oils. *Consumers' Research Magazine,* March.

Lee, A., et al. 2000. Consumption of tomato products with olive oil but not sunflower oil increases the antioxidant activity of plasma. *Free Radical Biology & Medicine* 29: 1051–1055.

Massaro, M., 1999. Direct vascular antiatherogenic effects of oleic acid: a clue to the cardioprotective effects of the Mediterranean diet. *Cardiologia* 44: 507–513.

McDonald, B. E. 2001. Canola oil: nutritional properties. Online: www.canola-council.org.

McGrath, M. 1999. How healthy is your olive oil? *Prevention,* September, pp. 122–127.

Newmark, H. L. 1997. Squalene, olive oil, and cancer risk: a review and hypothesis. *Cancer Epidemiology, Biomarkers & Prevention* 6: 1101–1103.

Nydahl, M., et al. 1995. Similar effects of rapeseed oil (canola oil) and olive oil in a lipid-lowering diet for patients with hyperlipoproteinemia. *Journal of the American College of Nutrition* 14: 643–651.

Ragionie, F. D., et al. 2000. Hyroxytyrosol, a natural molecule occurring in olive oil, induces cytochrome c-dependent apoptosis. *Biochemical and Biophysical Research Communications* 278: 733–739.

Ramirez-Tortosa, M. C., et al. 1999. Extra-virgin olive oil increases the resistance of LDL to oxidation more than refined olive oil in free-living men with peripheral vascular disease. *Journal of Nutrition* 129: 2177–2183.

Rodriguez-Villar, C., et al. 2000. High-monounsaturated fat, olive oil–rich diet has effects similar to a high-carbohydrate diet on fasting and postprandial state and metabolic profiles of patients with type 2 diabetes. *Metabolism* 49: 1511–1517.

Smith, T. J. 2000. Squalene: potential chemopreventive agent. *Expert Opinion on Investigational Drugs* 9: 1841–1848.

Trichopoulou, A., et al. 2000. Cancer and Mediterranean dietary traditions. *Cancer Epidemiology, Biomarkers & Prevention* 9: 869–873.

Visioli, F., et al. 1998. Free radical–scavenging properties of olive oil polyphenols. *Biochemical and Biophysical Research Communications* 9: 60–64.

Visioli, F., et al. 2000. Olive phenol hydroxytyrosol prevents passive smoking–induced oxidative stress. *Circulation* 102: 2169–2171.

Weil, A. 2000. What's the best olive oil? Ask Dr. Weil, June 6. Online: www.drweil.com.

Zambon, A., et al. 1999. Effects of hypocaloric dietary treatment enriched in oleic acid on LDL and HDL, subclass distribution in mildly obese women. *Journal of Internal Medicine* 246: 191–201.

Chapter 8. The New Heart-Saving Fats

American Dietetic Association. 1998. Fat replacers. Position statement. *Journal of the American Dietetic Association* 98: 463–468.

American Dietetic Association. 1995. Position of the American Dietetic Association: phytochemicals and functional foods. *Journal of the American Dietetic Association* 95: 493–496.

Blair, S. N. 2000. Incremental reduction of serum total cholesterol and low-density lipoprotein cholesterol with the addition of plant stanol ester-containing spread to statin therapy. *American Journal of Cardiology* 86: 46–52.

Editor. 2000. Can the new plant-based spreads really lower cholesterol? *John Hopkins Medical Letter Health After 50* 12: 98.

Gorman, C. 1999. It sure ain't butter. *Time,* May 31, p. 104.

Gylling, H., et al. 1997. Reduction of serum cholesterol in postmenopausal women with previous myocardial infarction and cholesterol malabsorption induced by dietary sitostanol ester margarine. *Circulation* 96: 4226–4231.

Hallikainen, M. A., et al. 1999. Effects of 2 low-fat stanol ester-containing margarines on serum cholesterol concentrations as part of a low-fat diet in hypercholesterolemic subjects. *American Journal of Clinical Nutrition* 69: 403–410.

Kulman, L. 1999. I really can believe it's not butter. *U.S. News & World Report,* May 31, p. 77.

Lipton. 2001. Take Control. Online: www.takecontrol.com.

McCord, H. 1999. Spread your bread. Help your heart. *Prevention*, October, p. 55.

McNeil Consumer Healthcare. 2001. Benecol. Online: www.benecol.com.

Miettinen, T. A., et al. 1995. Reduction of serum cholesterol with sitostanol-ester margarine in a mildly hypercholesterolemic population. *New England Journal of Medicine* 333: 1350–1351.

Plat, J., et al. 2000. Therapeutic potential of plat sterols and stanols. *Current Opinion in Lipidology* 11: 571–576.

Rosenthal, R. L. 2000. Effectiveness of altering serum cholesterol levels without drugs. *BUMC Proceedings* 13: 351–355.

Weststrate, J. A., et al. Plant sterol-enriched margarines and the reduction of plasma total and LDL cholesterol concentrations in normocholesterolaemic and mildly hypercholesterolaemic subjects. *European Journal of Clinical Nutrition* 52: 334–343.

Chapter 9. Conjugated Linoleic Acid: Health Insurance in a Pill

American Cancer Society. 2001. Statistics. Online: www.cancer.org.

American Heart Association. 2001. *2001 Heart and Stroke Statistical Update.* American Heart Association: Dallas, Texas, p. 4.

American Society of Bariatric Physicians. 2000. What is obesity? Online: www.asbp.org/obesity.htm.

Basu, S., et al. 2000. Conjugated linoleic acid induces lipid peroxidation in humans. *FEBS Letter* 468: 33–36.

Cesano, A., et al. 1998. Opposite effects of linoleic acid and conjugated linoleic acid on human prostatic cancer in SCID mice. *Anticancer Research* 18: 1429–1434.

Editor. 1996. Compounds in milk may reduce early indicators of cancer. *Cancer Weekly Plus,* November 11, 8.

Editor. 2001. Conjugated linoleic acid overview. Professional Monographs: Herbal, Mineral, Vitamin, Nutraceuticals. Intramedicine, March 1.

Editor. 2001. The dangerous toll of diabetes. Online: American Diabetes Association: www.diabetes.org.

Editor. 1996. Drinking milk regularly may cut risk of breast cancer. *Cancer Weekly Plus,* November 4, 22–23.

Editor. 2001. Raw material research: Tonalin® conjugated linoleic acid. *Nutraceuticals World* 4: 121.

Hayek, M. G., et al. 1999. Dietary conjugated linoleic acid influences the immune response of young and old C57BL/6NCrlBR mice. *Journal of Nutrition* 129: 32–38.

Houseknecht, K. L., et al. 1998. Dietary conjugated linoleic acid normalizes impaired glucose tolerance in the Zucker diabetic fatty fa/fa rat. *Biochemical and Biophysical Research Communications* 244: 678–682.

Kalman, D. S. 1998. Analyzing the latest natural weight loss supplements. *Muscular Development,* July, 96–98, 152–153.

Kreider, R., et al. Effects of conjugated linoleic acid (CLA) supplementation during resistance training on bone mineral content, bone mineral density, and markers of immune stress. *FASEB Journal* 4: A244.

Liu, K. L., et al. 1997. Conjugated linoleic acid modulation of phorbol ester-induced events in murine keratinocytes." *Lipids* 32: 725–730.

MacDonald, H. B. 2000. Conjugated linoleic acid and disease prevention: a review of current knowledge." *Journal of the American College of Nutrition* 19: 111S–118S.

Moya-Camarena, S. Y., et al. 1999. Species differences in the metabolism and regulation of gene expression by conjugated linoleic acid." *Nutrition Review* 57: 336–340.

Nature's Own. Conjugated linoleic acid. Internet Web address: www.naturesownusa.com/CLA.html.

Nicolosi, R. J., et al. 1997. Dietary conjugated linoleic acid reduces plasma lipoproteins and early aortic atherosclerosis in hypercholesterolemic hamsters. *Artery* 22: 266–277.

Pariza, M. W., et al. Mechanisms of action of conjugated linoleic acid; evidence and speculation. *Proceedings of the Society for Experimental Biology and Medicine* 223: 8–13.

Parodi, P. W. 1997. Cows' milk fat components as potential anticarcinogenic agents. *Journal of Nutrition* 127: 1055–1060.

Raloff, J. 1994. This fat may fight cancer several ways. *Science News* 145: 182–183.

Schechter, S. 1997. Fat intake can boost weight loss, if we are selective about our choices. *Better Nutrition,* June, 26.

Truitt, A., et al. 1999. Antiplatelet effects of conjugated linoleic acid isomers. *Biochimica et Biophysica Acta* 1438: 239–246.

Tsuboyama-Kasaoka, N. 2000. Conjugated linoleic acid supplementation reduces adipose tissue by apoptosis and develops lipodystrophy in Mice. *Diabetes Care* 49: 1534–1542.

West, D. B., et al. 1998. Effects of conjugated linoleic acid on body fat and energy metabolism in the mouse. *American Journal of Physiology* 275: R667–R672.

Chapter 10. MCT Oil: The Dieter's Fat

Calabrese, et al. 1999. A cross-over study of the effect of a single oral feeding of medium chain triglyceride oil vs. canola oil on post-ingestion plasma triglyceride levels in healthy men. *Alternative Medicine Review* 4:23–26.

Dias, V. 1990. Effects of feeding and energy balance in adult humans. *Metabolism* 39: 887–891.

Dulloo, A. G., M. Fathi, N. Mensi, and L. Girardier. 1996. Twenty-four-hour energy expenditure and urinary catecholamines of humans consuming low-to-moderate amounts of medium-chain triglycerides: a dose-response study in a human respiratory chamber. *European Journal of Clinical Nutrition* 50: 152–158

Editor. 1993. Good nutrition can help athletes lose weight. *Better Nutrition* 55: 22–23.

Editor. 1995. MCT oil. *Environmental Nutrition* 8: 7.

Hainer, V., et al. 1994. The role of oils containing triacylglycerols and medium-chain fatty acids in the dietary treatment of obesity. The effect on resting energy expenditure and serum lipids. *Casopis Lekaru Ceskych* 133: 373–375.

Hill, J. O., J. C. Peters, D. Yang, et al. 1989. Thermogenesis in humans during overfeeding with medium-chain triglycerides. *Metabolism* 38: 641–648.

Roberson, A., and Parrillo, J. 1997. *Medium-chain triglycerides in sports.* Cincinnati, Ohio: Parrillo Performance.

Seaton, T. B., S. L. Welle, M. K. Warenko, and R. G. Campbell. 1986. Thermic effect of medium- and long-chain triglycerides in man. *American Journal of Clinical Nutrition* 44: 630–634.

Stubbs, R. J., and C. G. Harbon. 1996. Covert manipulation of the ratio of medium- to long-chain triglycerides in isoenergetically dense diets: effect on food intake in ad libitum feeding men. *International Journal of Eating Disorders* 20: 435–444.

Traul, K. A., et al. 2000. Review of toxicologic properties of medium-chain triglycerides. *Food and Chemical Toxicology 38: 79–98.*

Van Zyl, C. 1996. Effects of medium chain triglyceride ingestion on fuel metabolism and cycling performance. *Journal of Applied Psychology* 80:2217–2225.

Chapter 11. A Smart-Fat Strategy

American Heart Association. 2001. Heart and stroke guide. Online: www.americanheart.org.

Kris-Etherton, P. M. 2000. Polyunsaturated fatty acids in the food chain in the United States. *American Journal of Clinical Nutrition* 71: 179–188.

Reuters Health. 2000. Studies suggest Atkins diet is safe. Online: www.heartinfo.org.

Webb, D. 1999. Healthy diet: the smart fat makeover. *Prevention,* April, pp. 134–141.

Chapter 12. Good Fat Cooking

Crowley, M. B. 1998. Dressing up with oil. *Chatelaine,* October, p. 212D.

About the Author

Maggie Greenwood-Robinson, Ph.D., is one of the country's top health and medical authors. She is the author of *Wrinkle-Free: Your Guide to Youthful Skin at Any Age*, *The Bone Density Test*, *Hair Savers for Women: A Complete Guide to Preventing and Treating Hair Loss*, *The Cellulite Breakthrough*, *Natural Weight Loss Miracles*, *Kava: The Ultimate Guide to Nature's Anti-Stress Herb*, and *21 Days to Better Fitness*. She is also the coauthor of nine other fitness books, including the national bestseller *Lean Bodies*, *Lean Bodies Total Fitness*, *High Performance Nutrition*, *Power Eating*, and *50 Workout Secrets*.

Her articles have appeared in *Let's Live*, *Physical Magazine*, *Great Life*, *Shape Magazine*, *Christian Single Magazine*, *Women's Sports and Fitness*, *Working Woman*, *Muscle and Fitness*, *Female Bodybuilding and Fitness*, and many other publications. She is a member of the advisory board of *Physical Magazine*. In additon, she has a doctorate in nutritional counseling and is a certified nutritional consultant.